SOTHIS PRESS

Sothis Press aims to completely reimagine the public domain book with an emphasis on universal access to captivatingly designed print editions. We believe that technology will enable every single book ever published to be perpetually accessible in beautiful print form. Sothis is beauty in ubiquity.

www.sothis.press
1 Waterhouse Square, London, ECIN 2ST

Nerve-Vibration and Excitation as Agents in the Treatment of Functional Disorder and Organic Disease

J. Mortimer Granville

SOTHIS PRESS

ISBN 978-1-0365-1620-8

Nerve-Vibration and Excitation as Agents in the Treatment of Functional Disorder and Organic Disease is in the public domain.

NERVE-VIBRATION AND EXCITATION

AS

AGENTS IN THE TREATMENT OF FUNCTIONAL DISORDER AND ORGANIC DISEASE.

BY

J. MORTIMER GRANVILLE, M.D.

LONDON:
J. & A. CHURCHILL,
NEW BURLINGTON STREET.
1883.

TO THE READER.

THE time has arrived when it seems incumbent upon me to place before the profession in a succinct form my views on the subject of nerve-vibration and excitation as remedial agents, or processes, for the treatment of functional disorder and organic disease.

I publish the statements submitted in the following pages in the spirit of an investigator who feels bound to report the progress he has made in an arduous and difficult inquiry. It will be only fair to understand that the *inferences* I have drawn from a large, though perhaps insufficient, series of clinical observations, are held and put forth tentatively. Further experience may necessitate both corrections and recantations. Meanwhile, of the matters I have treated as *facts* in this little treatise I am assured. It is only as to their significance, and the relative value which should be attached to them, there can be any question.

I ask nothing more than that courteous hearing which is commonly accorded to the explorer who announces the discovery of a new province, and such confidence as may induce others to help in the investigation of what seems likely to prove an important addition to the number and range of our remedial resources.

J. MORTIMER GRANVILLE.

16, WELBECK STREET.

CONTENTS.

INTRODUCTORY.

I DO not affirm that nervous force is the product of nerve-vibration ; but science certainly justifies the belief that nerve action, or activity, consists in, or is accompanied by, vibrations of the essential elements of nervous tissue in the body, or frame—so to say—formed by the complementary parts of its structure.

Cells vibrate as bodies suspended in the intercellular stroma of the grey matter, and fibres vibrate as delicately poised rods or strung cords within the partite cylinders formed by internal prolongations of the neurilemma or nerve sheath.

When deposits take place, in the progress of disease, in the interstices of a nervous cell bed, or between, or upon, the layers or partition walls of a nerve sheath, or when the connective tissue forming the framework of a nervous structure proliferates, the vibration of cell or fibre is mechanically prevented, and the discharge or transmission of nervous force from a centre or along a nerve becomes physically impracticable.

The pathological anatomist calls this solidification of the stroma of the nervous organism sclerosis, and thinks that in it he has found the efficient *cause* of loss of sensation or deprivation of power. He accepts the *post hoc*, and interprets it as the *propter hoc*. In all humility, I venture to doubt the accuracy of his judgment, and to dispute the logical character of his reasoning. It is, I think, by no means certain that sclerosis of the posterior or anterior columns of the spinal cord is the *cause* of anæsthesia or of myo-paralysis respectively. If the student of morbid appearances in the nervous system will take the trouble to examine even a small area of sclerosed brain, cord, or nerve tissue, carefully, particularly in the most recent zones or tracts marking the progress of the disease, he will almost certainly find some, often many, cells or fibres which lie atrophied amid their surroundings, with clear interspaces between their shrivelled walls, and the adventitious matter producing the sclerosis. In short, solidification, or sclerosis, is not less likely to be the consequence or concomitant of atrophy of the essential elements of nervous tissue than to be its cause.

The significance of this alternative reading of the record left by disease in the post-mortem appearances will be obvious, when we reflect that if cell and fibre are the parts of nervous structure which first suffer in the advances of paralytic disease, and the sclerosis is contingent and secondary, it may well happen, if, indeed, it be not probable, that by an energetic and wise application of the law of development by exercise, the nutrition of the nervous elements may be improved, and their recovery effected by stimulation through function. If the degenerating, but, perhaps, not yet irrecoverably degenerated, cells or fibres are thrown into vibration they may act, and, in obedience to the law which determines that every particle of organic matter shall feed as it works and in that proportion only, they may begin to take in increased nourishment, and recover in virtue of the *vis medicatrix* of the organism as they are healthily stimulated by rhythmical motion. Moreover, by inducing and maintaining vibratile movements in the nervous elements proper, the encroachment of the solidifying deposit or proliferating connective tissue may be arrested, the mere mechanical motion of the nerve structure tending to shake the elements loose from any recent and as yet unconsolidated entanglement, and to promote the absorption of adventitious material, in such manner as the thickening around a joint, or those adhesive bands which spring up within or between tendons and their sheaths, are broken down and ultimately absorbed under the influence of passive movements. Whatever else we may do to promote the absorption of deposits, our first aim should be to restore or preserve the free mobility of the vibratile elements, and in no other way can this be so readily or effectively accomplished as by mechanical vibration.

I do not think the mechanical vibration of nerve tissue can be effected by electricity, or, at least, with the constant current. That current simply uses the nerve structure as a conductor, and passes along it without throwing it into vibration. Electricity travels in the line of least resistance, without relation to the particular tissue which offers itself as a conductor, except so far as regards its capacity for receiving and transmitting the current. Electricity will pass along the track of a nerve, taking the place of nervous energy, and itself producing the phenomena of muscular contraction instead of eliciting nervous force from the nerve centres. So far as the nutrition of tissues other than the nervous, is concerned, the value of constant, or static, electricity is beyond question. It is one of the most potent therapeutic agents we possess, and when intelligently and expertly applied, signally useful; but I do not think it improves the nutrition of the nerve or nerve centres, unless it be indirectly. The interrupted current acts differently. This has the power of throwing any particle of matter, whether living or inorganic, into mechanical vibration, and it is, therefore, quite possible that it may throw nerve elements into vibration, but if it does, there is added to this good the doubtful effect of infusing the organism with a force which is foreign to its economy, although it may closely resemble the nervous force it substitutes. By introducing an electric current into the body, we are taking the function of activity out of the hands of Nature, and throwing the proper function of the nerve elements into abeyance; whereas, by simply calling out nervous force from the nerve centres, by throwing them and their interconnecting fibres into vibration, we are waiting on Nature, and helping her to do her work with her own forces and in her own way. All that is done by the nervous system in respect to the stimulus of vibration is necessarily performed by nervous force, elicited, reflexly, from the nerve centres. It cannot be otherwise, because mere vibration has nothing to communicate beyond its own "form of motion."

The facts underlying the principle of nerve-vibration and excitation by mechanical movement may be set out as follows:—

1. When nervous tissue acts, its essential elements—viz., cells and fibres—vibrate. It follows that by throwing these elements into vibration by mechanical movement, we establish a condition favourable to the discharge of nervous force from the centres affected, and at the same time stimulate the nerve centre, when discharged, to develop new force to compensate the loss of energy expended in exercise.

2. The vibration of nervous elements being a purely mechanical process, it must be conformable to the laws or conditions that govern the vibratile movement of other bodies, whether organic or inorganic—for example, reed instruments—and the vibration of cells and fibres should, therefore, be amenable to the laws of concord and discord. In short, what Newton discovered and taught in explication of the phenomena of light and sound, with the recognized correlations of the diatonic and chromatic scales, must be equally applicable to an as yet unrecognized but doubtless existing scale of nerve-vibrations. And such affinity must exist between the nature of the faculty, and the working of the organic apparatus, of perception, in regard to sound, colour, and other forms or properties of the external, and other physical processes whereby these forms or properties of matter are produced, that the nervous system and the external world are not simply *en rapport*, but physically correlated. It is, therefore, only reasonable to suppose that the evolution of nervous force is governed by the same laws that govern the evolution (or production) of light, colour, sound, odour, and other qualities or properties of matter which are in many instances demonstrably, and

in all others presumably, due to modes and formulæ of mechanical vibration. For example, light and sound are effects of the specific vibration of particles or molecules of matter, and they produce their characteristic phenomena (so far as we are cognisant of their existence), by vibrating the special apparatus of the eye and the ear respectively—namely, the rod and cones of the retina in the eye, and the loops or terminal expansion of the auditory nerve in the internal ear. These several sets of mechanical vibrations are propagated along the fibres of the second and seventh nerves to their respective centres, wherein, by the vibration of cells, in mechanical relation with the communicating nerves, the function of special perception is performed.

3. As a necessary result of this state of matters, it must be possible to act on the nervous system by purely mechanical agents and influences, with the effect of interrupting, modifying, or altogether arresting organic vibrations, whether in afferent sensory or efferent motor nerves. These effects are capable of demonstration, producing changes in the rate and rhythm of nerve vibration precisely correspondent with those which would be effected in the vibration of unorganized substances by the operation of the same or similar agents working in like processes.

The system or method of treatment which I am anxious to bring under the very serious consideration of the profession consists in the application of the laws of physical, or mechanical, vibration as they affect ordinary substances, to the interruption and change of morbid states of the vibratile organism. The apparatus by which the desired movements are produced is altogether secondary in importance to the principle itself. I use percussion ; others may use vibratory instruments which do not percuss the tissue, but communicate their own vibrations to the organism by simple continuity. This I take to be the method adopted by M. Boudet de Paris, who more than two years after my percuteurs were in the hands of leading physiologists and therapeutists, published a paper in *Le Progrès Médical*, wherein he set forth views and described a method differing in several important particulars from my own, but practically embodying the same idea. *The Lancet*, of Feb. 12, 1881, just four years after my instruments were made in London, contained the following summary of M. Boudet de Paris' paper :—

"TREATMENT OF PAIN BY MECHANICAL VIBRATIONS.

"For some years past Dr. Mortimer Granville has been occupied with important researches upon the possibility of combating neuralgia by mechanical means. Proceeding largely upon theoretical considerations, he came to the conclusion that a series of interrupted mechanical shocks to a nerve would diminish its sensibility, and for that purpose invented a small instrument whereby a succession of rapid blows could be kept up upon the skin. Many physicians in London and Paris have seen and employed the apparatus, and spoken of it with approval ; but Dr. Granville forbore to bring it under general notice until it had been thoroughly tested. He has paid the penalty of his patience, and the old story is repeated of the publication of an idea by another person by whom it was conceived long after the one who first thought of it, but who did not proclaim it to the world. In justice to himself, Dr. Granville should forthwith point out how he arrived at the idea, and state his experience of its practical enforcement. Meanwhile it may be interesting to summarize the statements of M. Boudet de Paris, who writes on the subject in the current number of *Le Progrès Médical*. After alluding to Dr. Brown-Séquard's observation that chloroform applied over the skin of an animal produces general anæsthesia by its irritant action on the peripheral nerves, he points out that all irritants or revulsives may be placed in one category—such as actual cautery, hypodermic injections of water, application of metals, magnets, tuning-forks, electricity, vesicatories, sinapisms, compresses steeped in ether or chloroform, a motley group, but each intended for the same end—the relief of pain; they all operate by irritating the terminal twigs of sensory nerves. Vulpian long ago showed the good effect of the local application of chloroform; and Landouzy has recently pointed out the remarkable influence in controlling the cough of phthisis by hypodermic injections of water; whilst the cautery, acupuncture, and each of the forms of electricity are commonly applied to relieve pain. The action of metallic applications—metallo-therapy—of which we have heard so much in the last few years, was best explained on the theory of vibrations by Vigouroux, who proceeded to experiment upon the effect of sonorous vibrations, which he thought might have a direct mechanical effect upon the sensory nerves. By the aid of a large tuning fork and sounding-board he caused hemianæsthesia to disappear, and provoked contractions in hysterical subjects at la Salpétrière, as rapidly as with the magnet or electricity. The pains of an ataxic were subdued when his legs were brought under the influence of these sound-waves. M. Boudet de Paris then thought this might be applied locally over a nerve—the sonorous being changed to mechanical vibrations by means of a small button attached to the resonater, and applied over the nerve. He therefore contrived a small apparatus consisting of an electrically mounted tuning fork, the vibrations of which were transmitted to a rod which could be easily applied over a nerve. In a healthy man this mechanical excitation produced rapid local analgesia, often anæsthesia, the maximum effect being produced by application over a nerve which could be compressed on a bony surface. When placed against the skull its walls vibrate in harmony with the tuning-fork, and a sensation of approaching vertigo, frequently followed by a desire for sleep, is produced. An attack of migraine can be cut short by the application. Neuralgia—especially of the fifth, where the nerves issue from bony canals—disappears after a few minutes' application of the instrument to the nerve at such points, but in the case of deeper-seated nerves, much protected by soft parts, it is more difficult to get good results. The writer suggests this treatment for the pains of ataxics and syphilitics ; he thinks there is no limit to its applications, and suggests that perhaps cranial vibrations may induce cerebral and thus general anæsthesia. Its mechanical action is comprehensible, when we see how simple friction of the skin may soothe very acute pain. He does not regard the number of vibrations as important. This, however, is we believe, a point on which Dr. Mortimer Granville lays the greatest stress." The publication of this paper by M. Boudet de Paris, describing the method of M. Vigouroux, forced my hand, so to say, and compelled me to place the results of many years study of the subject prematurely before the profession. My investigations grew out of a search for means to relieve the intolerable pain of neuralgia. It will be convenient to reproduce my own paper, which appeared in *The Lancet*, February 19, 1881, as it is virtually a reply to M. Boudet de Paris :—

"The publication of certain results obtained in an investigation which I have been pursuing for some years past, having been to a large extent anticipated by a paper which appeared in *Le Progrès Médical* of the 5th inst., from the pen of M. Boudet de Paris, ancien interne des hôpitaux de Paris, I have no alternative but to bring my researches, together with such facts, real or imaginary, as I have succeeded in eliciting, under the notice of the profession here and on the Continent, Indeed, I owe some explanation to many friends in England and in Paris for having so long delayed to report the progress of my experiments. Nevertheless I break silence thus early with the greatest reluctance, and only under the pressure of circumstances. As regards the accident of 'forestalling,' if I am not mistaken, M. Boudet de Paris will have greater cause than I have to regret what I cannot but feel is the premature announcement of a discovery. On August 5, 1878, Professor Brown-Séquard wrote me as follows:—'If it (the instrument employed in these experiments) has the power you state, you have certainly made a very important discovery.' I could not but feel that there was a virtue in that 'if' to enforce reserve until other judgments besides my own were fully satisfied. Such grave responsibility attaches to any member of the profession who ventures to suggest a new, or seemingly new, method of treatment, and who dares to hold out a hope of remedy or relief for the miseries of mankind, that I, for one, must confess to a great shrinking from the hazard of rushing into print prematurely. This feeling alone has induced me to keep silence during the last three or four years, and I am convinced the same motive has influenced the several physicians who have kindly tried my method and employed my percuteur, to wait until convinced of their validity and value before giving to either the sanction of their authority. Among the gentlemen to whom I have submitted my speculations, and shown my instrument, I may mention Professor Brown-Séquard, Professor Ball, and Dr. Oscar Jennings of Paris, and Drs. Ringer and Gowers of London. These names are in themselves sufficient to guarantee that, if the results obtained by experiment had been such as to establish my conclusions, they would long since have been announced, and, unless I am greatly mistaken, the results recorded by M. Boudet de Paris cannot, in any therapeutical sense, be more trustworthy than my own. I will now tell the story of my investigations, and thus mark the point reached in the search for a new remedy.

"As far back as 1862-3, I was, in the course of certain clinical studies of mental and sensory phenomena, induced to believe that many forms of the sensation we call 'pain' were in fact, unnecessary, and might be *interrupted* by appropriate mental and physical methods and appliances. My first observations were made in connection with the paroxysmal, or recurrent, pains accompanying the uterine contractions in the natural process of parturition. On May 4, 1864, Dr. Graily Hewitt was good enough to communicate the results of my experiments and to show certain apparatus to the Obstetrical Society of London. In a paper 'On the Application of Extreme Cold as an Anodyne in the Pain attendant on Parturition,' a short abstract of which will be found in *The Lancet* of July 9, 1864, I contended that the sensations of pain experienced by the parturient woman were not invariably synchronous with what, for want of a better name, we term the pains of labour ; and from this and other premisses—for example, the circumstance that they are commonly 'referred' to regions more or less remote from the contracting uterus, or the dilating external passages, in which the real seat of the pain might have been supposed to be located—I deduced that the pain attendant on labour is *neuralgic* in character. I had constructed small boxes or chambers of such sizes and shapes as to admit of their being applied to the *supposed* seats of the pain. These were filled with freezing mixture, and the effect of sudden contact in some thirty cases was to arrest the sensation of pain without in the least degree lessening the force of the uterine contractions. The experiment was of course simply interesting as bearing on the nature of the pain, as this process was too troublesome to admit of its adoption in practice; although some of the persons on whom I had the opportunity of trying my method experienced such striking relief that on subsequent occasions I believe they asked that the measure might be repeated. Having so far persuaded myself that this form of pain was neuralgic, and that if the nerve affected could be strongly impressed, so as to change its state of irritation, the pain would cease, I proceeded to try the effect of rapidly tapping the skin over the fifth nerve in ordinary facial neuralgia with a Bennett's percussion hammer, using the ivory pleximeter as a shield. The results obtained by this method were very remarkable. Still, I simply thought of arresting the morbid action by *shock*. Later on—it is only possible to sketch the outline of the inquiry—I was led, by the light thrown on Newton's doctrine of concords and discords, by Grove's generalization as to the correlation of forces, and more recently by Professor Tyndall's beautiful series of experiments with sensitive flames and musical burners, to believe that the results of the tapping were not, like the interruption with shock produced by the sudden application of cold, due to a mere arrest of the painful state of irritation into which the nerve had been thrown, but were, in fact, brought about by the extinguishment of a morbid—that is, either inordinate or disorderly—set of vibrations by the super-imposition of another, incompatible or discordant, set of vibrations mechanically produced. With this notion I set to work to devise an instrument which should give a known number of blows per second, and thus admit of this new phase of the inquiry being pushed farther. Such an instrument was made for me at the establishment of Mr. Streeter, of New Bond Street, from a sketch and specification dated January 5, 1877. With the 'percuteur' thus made, and others by M. Collin, of Paris, results which I would characterize as suggestive rather than conclusive have certainly been obtained, They are, in brief, as follows :—

"The sensation produced by the application of the instrument over a healthy nerve, so situated as to be readily thrown into mechanical vibration, closely resembles the effect of a weak dose of the interrupted current of electricity, and if it be prolonged the vibration extends its area, exciting first formication or tingling, then a sensation of numbness, and finally some twitching of the superficial muscles. A nervous headache, and even migraine, may be induced by the application of the percuteur to the frontal ridges or the margins of the orbit. By the intervention of a thin plate of metal, or stiff paper, the vibration may be readily propagated through a considerable region of the surface of the body, and in time the deeper muscles will frequently begin to act. I have, indeed, produced an involuntary movement, not unlike tendon-reflex, by applying the percuteur for some time over the tendon of the rectus femoris *above* the patella. Still more notable has been the fact that by laying a sheet of paper over the abdomen, and moving the percuteur slowly in large circles round the umbilicus, the intestines have seemed to be excited to vermicular movement, and the bowels commenced to act. These results have not been constant, but have occurred with sufficient frequency to indicate that the experiments already made are worthy to be repeated.

"With respect to the relief of neuralgic pain, the operations of the instrument are certainly very remarkable, but not, in my judgment or in that of other observers, such as to justify the assertion that it constitutes an appliance for the relief of pain. In some instances —pretty numerous—the pain of neuralgia in the branches of the fifth has been quickly arrested by its application, and has not soon returned, or, if it has done so, has again unmistakably yielded. In other instances the sensation has been aggravated by the augmented state of vibration into which the nerve has been thrown through the shaking of the adjacent tissues. And here I must mention a point to which I attach the greatest moment, and which, I think, will hereafter be found to prove the key to the whole phenomena. A comparatively high number of vibrations per second seems to relieve a dull aching, a 'massive' or grinding pain, while an acutely pitched and quick pain is most frequently arrested by a slower movement of the instrument. If I may step beyond the province of a simple reporter of clinical phenomena for one moment, I will take leave to say that I think these results go to support my theory that it is by the introduction of *discord* into the rhythm of the morbid vibrations of the painful 'state' the change which brings relief is effected.

To apply the percuteur with a high rate of blows per second will aggravate the morbid state when that is itself a series of rapid vibrations, and in the same way a low speed of percussion increases, instead of relieving, the pains of a low pitched and slow 'boring' or 'grinding' sensation. Acute or sharp pain is, I believe, like a high note in music, produced by rapid vibrations, while a dull, heavy, or aching pain resembles a low note or tone, and is caused by comparatively slow vibrations. A slow rate of mechanical vibration will therefore interrupt the rapid nerve-vibration of acute pain, while quick mechanical vibration more readily arrests the slower. The aim—if I am right in my conjecture—should be to set up a new set of vibrations which shall interrupt or change the morbid set by introducing discord. Failure in the application of this principle will, I believe, be found to explain the failure to put an end to the pain; and I have, accordingly, set as much scientific value on my failures as on my successes.

"My percuteurs are all defective in one particular: although they consist of a simple train of cogged-wheels worked by a spring and acting on a lever which carries an ivory hammer, and are provided with an indicator, which shows the speed, and a screw movement to control it, they do not obey the will of the operator, because the slightest pressure of his hand shortens the arc in which the hammer works, and proportionally accelerates the stroke. M. Collin has modified my instrument, but he has not, so far as I am aware, entirely remedied this defect. If M. Boudet de Paris can so improve his instrument as to obtain control of its movements and to propagate a *known* set of vibrations, he may succeed better than I have done; but I should be glad to find that the result could be obtained without the use of electricity, as it is important to the scientific interest of the instrument—and as yet it cannot, I am convinced, be said to have a therapeutic value—to show that the vibrations are purely mechanical, and propagated through the tissues by a force acting externally. It would be one thing to induce change of the organic vibrations by internal force, and quite another to overpower the internal movements by force operating from without. The result may be the same, but the two methods of reaching it are essentially different.

"That all nerve action is vibratile, and that the neuralgic state consists essentially in an abnormal set or series of vibrations into which the nerve has been thrown —perhaps by a jet of cold air, or a mechanical or chemical irritant—I have no doubt. That this state may be changed by mechanical vibrations propagated to the nerve-sheath and its contents through the adjacent tissues I am convinced. I have not, however, as yet, got one step further than persuading myself that these are genuine propositions, and capable of demonstration by experiment—to wit, the causation of neuralgic pain, and the induction of the neuralgic state generally, by mechanical vibrations, and the relief of these conditions, when they exist, by the same method. The essence of the process is disturbance and change of the rhythm. When I began to study the effect of cold, I thought the results obtained were reached by deadening the nerve or 'lowering its sensibility,' as we say; but I soon found that the effect was proportioned to the intensity of the shock produced by the sudden contact with the cold substance, not the duration of the chilling process. When cold gives relief by its continuance, rather than instantly on its application, I think that is because the morbid vibrations of the nerve cannot, for some physical reason, be interrupted by shock; possibly the nerve is situated too deeply, or is covered by dense tissues, or lies so loosely amid its surroundings as to be practically insulated, and the morbid vibrations are not arrested until the cold contracts the surrounding tissues, and causes them to mechanically grip the terminal twigs of the nerve which is vibrating painfully. In some instances the percuteur is so powerful as to arrest the morbid vibrations on one side and propagate a painful set of vibrations through the centre to the other side. This may strike the reader as a mere assertion, but I am persuaded it will be found to be borne out by experiment. If I am not greatly mistaken, the percuteur, or some more perfect mechanical vibrator, will do all that 'metallo-therapy' has achieved in the same class of cases. We do not sufficiently appreciate the effect of subtle or subtilly applied forces acting on the organism. When the so-called mesmerist induces a state of hypnotism in his patient by simply blowing on the face, or when by 'passes' he impresses the retina, he acts *physically* on the terminal twigs of highly sensitive —and generally educated—nerves, and induces a set of actions which, though notable in themselves, are no more mysterious in the manner of their production than the involuntary strong muscular action excited by the 'tickling' of a hair or a feather, or the crawling of an insect. As a matter of fact, the surface is generally more powerfully impressed by these minor applications of mechanical force than by the greater. If you touch an exposed sub-cuticular surface lightly you give extreme pain ; if you grasp it somewhat firmly you cause less suffering. This is quite as likely to be because, in the first case, the terminal twigs of the sensitive nerves are set vibrating, whereas in the latter vibration is pre-prevented, as due to the local blood-change to which these results are commonly attributed. While a poultice is moist, and clings to the surface of a sore, it soothes by holding the nerve-fibres still ; when it begins to dry, and they are liberated, the poultice becomes an irritant. The physical basis of the so-called hysterical state, or the peculiarity of nervous organization which predisposes to hysteria, is, I think, simply a class or type of structure which renders the nervous elements especially liable to vibrate in their sheaths, and thus exposes them to the risk of falling readily into any rhythm which the will, the physico-mental environment, or perhaps even the proximity of similar structures vibrating in other bodies characterized by the same physical organization, may suggest. If musical burners, supplied from different reservoirs of gas, will presently vibrate in concord ; if strings or reeds vibrating at the same time, though a short distance apart, will fall into harmony, why is it unlikely that nervous organisms, possessing the same qualities of physical structure, should exhibit a corresponding affinity? Science points clearly to physical states, as the bases of nervous and mental phenomena. The female organism is characterized not inaccurately, though popularly, by the phrase 'finely strung nerves.' It is literally *mobile*, and it is chiefly among females the phenomena of hysteria, and the allied states, are observed. When the symptoms and conditions so designated do occur in the male, the individual organism is generally of a feminine character.

"In conclusion, I would venture to predict that it will be found that nerve action, both normal and abnormal, consists of vibrations, and that other mechanical vibrations set up and propagated by any mechanical apparatus or appliance, acting from without and propagated through the tissues, may be made to modify the internal movements; that normal vibrations consist of movements of the constituent parts of a nerve within its sheath, and that when these become inordinate or disorderly they are propagated to the sheath itself, and then become painful; that under this last-mentioned condition the wave of vibration is likely to be propagated along the sheath of the nerve, and through it to the sheaths of other nerves with which the first in order of disturbance may be mechanically related, either by direct contact or through intervening tissues; that the action of irritants applied to the skin is mechanical, producing contraction of the tissues, and either first gripping and then relaxing the terminal twigs of the nerves, thus throwing them into mechanical vibration, or so changing the constitution of the bed in which these terminal twigs lie, as to oppose a mechanical obstruction to their natural vibration, and thereby convert it into a morbid rhythm. This, indeed, has been demonstrated by Dr. Ringer, in his classic treatise on Therapeutics, in connexion with the *modus operandi* of blisters, etc. These may be set down as crude speculations, but they are the results to which experiment and commonplace reasoning point, and they are in harmony with a view of the phenomena of nerve action and of pain which the inquiry I am pursuing forces upon me, and by which nearly all the wonders of the hysterical school of medical philosophy may be explained. I cannot claim to have discovered a 'cure' for neuralgia, or even a certain method of treatment for its relief. The time has not arrived when it may be possible to commend this new method to the notice of the medical profession as a known agency for the alleviation of suffering; but as the facts have been prematurely published, I think the method should be tried."

It will be noted that whereas M. Boudet de Paris does not, as *The Lancet* pointed out, attach any importance to the rate or rhythm of the mechanical vibrations wherewith he strives to interrupt the morbid and painful vibrations of the nerves on which he operates, I regard that point as of crucial moment, and believe the issue of success or failure will be mainly determined by the musical relation which exists between the externally induced motion and that which it is desired to control or arrest.

As to the question of priority, this was happily settled for me, at once, by the friendly promptitude of Professor Brown-Séquard, Professor Ball, and Dr. Oscar Jennings in Paris, and Dr. Sydney Ringer and others in London, to whom my percuteurs were submitted long before the experiments, upon which M. Boudet de Paris founded his paper, were undertaken. As a matter of fact, nerve-vibration by percussion, with instruments furnished by myself, was tried at the National Hospital in Queen Square, London, in January and February, 1878.

The following is a note furnished to me by one of the medical officers of the institution at that date:—

"A medical man complained of neuralgic pain in his right internal cutaneous nerve, resulting, as he supposed, from a blow by a cricket ball. The pain came on at varying intervals, and during the intervals he could produce it by squeezing the site of the blow. The application of the instrument entirely stopped the pain and, much to his surprise, for a few minutes after he was unable to reproduce it. These experiments were repeated twenty or thirty times with the same result."

The percuteur with which these experiments were performed, was made for me by Mr. Streeter, of New Bond Street, from drawings dated Jan. 5, 1877. Later on, but still long before the researches of M. Vigouroux and M. Boudet de Paris, my percuteurs were on trial at the Laënnec Hospital, and the hospital of St. Anne, by the courtesy of Professor Ball. Professor Brown-Séquard affirmed my claim to priority before the Biological Society of Paris; Professor Ball did the same in *L'Encéphale;* and Dr. Oscar Jennings addressed the following letter to *Le Progrès Médical,* calling forth the annexed rejoinder from M. Boudet de Paris:—

"TRAITEMENT DE LA DOULEUR PAR LES VIBRATIONS MÉCANIQUES.

" Nous avons reçu, à propos du travail de M. Boudet de Paris que nous avons publié il y quelques jours (1) la lettre suivante de M. le Dr. Jennings.

Monsieur le Rédacteur,—Dans un article qui a paru dans le dernier numéro du *Progrès Médical*, M. Boudet de Paris s'occupe du traitement mécanique de la douleur.

Longtemps avant votre collaborateur, un médecin anglais, M. le Dr. Mortimer-Granville, s'était occupé de la même question. Il a même inventé un instrument spécial qu'il a nommé 'le percuteur.' Cet instrument est destiné à frapper des coups redoublés sur la partie malade, avec une rapidité que l'on peut graduer à volonté. Il se vend chez Collin, le successeur de Charrière. M. Granville a fait l'essai de son instrument à Londres, il y a quatre ans, et des essais suivis ont eu lieu l'année dernière dans le service de M. le Professeur Ball, à l'hôpital Laënnec. Je possède de nombreuses observations qui permettent d'apprécier la valeur de ce traitement. Si elles n'ont pas été publiées jusqu'à présent, c'est parce que l'utilité pratique du percuteur ne me paraissait pas suffisamment démontrée. Il calme incontestablement la douleur, mais pour un temps limité. Cette observation s'appliquerait peut-être aux moyens employés par M. Boudet de Paris. En tout cas, on ne peut se dispenser de reconnaître les droits de priorité de mon ami M. Mortimer-Granville, à cet égard.

"Je viens vous prier, M. le Rédacteur, d'insérer cette

lettre dans un prochain numéro, et d'agréer l'assurance de ma parfaite consideration.

"Dr. OSCAR JENNINGS."

Notre collaborateur, auquel nous avons communiqué cette lettre, nous prie d'insérer la réponse suivante.

"Mon cher Rédacteur,—M. le Dr. Jennings réclame la priorité, pour le traitement mécanique de la douleur, au bénéfice du Dr. Mortimer-Granville. J'avoue ne pas bien saisir le motif pour lequel M. Jennings a senti la nécessité de mettre ma personnalité en avant. Dans l'article que vous avez bien voulu publier, j'ai rapporté les expériences du Dr. Vigoureux sur les mystériques, décrit un moyen pratique de renouveler ces expériences au point de vue therapeutique, et, enfin, discuté l'action physiologique de la méthode. De la à une invention il y a loin. Je ne pensais pas, en écrivant cet article, que l'on pût me reprocher d'avoir pris quelque chose à quelqu'un. J'ai reconnu M. le Dr. Vigouroux comme le promoteur de l'idée d'employer le diapason. Je crois le fait indéniable, et, jusqu'à preuve du contraire, je resterai de cet avis.

"Les 'nombreuses observations inédites' que possède M. Jennings seront sans doute d'un grand intérêt en pareille occasion, mais il avouera que je ne pouvais pas supposer leur existence. Je n'insiste pas plus longtemps. Ni M. Mortimer-Granville, ni M. Jennings, ni M. Vigouroux, ni moi n'avons *inventé les vibrations.* M. Vigouroux, puis moi, en avons parlé, M. Jennings voudra bien reconnaître que c'était notre droit.

"Voilà, mon cher confrère, ce que je crois devoir répondre à la lettre, d'ailleurs fort courtoise, de M. Jennings ; je regrette seulement qu'il soit à peu près impossible d'écrire quelques lignes dans un journal scientifique, sans voir immédiatement surgir des réclamations de priorité.

"Veuillez agréer, etc.

"Dr. M. BOUDET DE PARIS."

There is no reason to suppose that either M. Vigouroux or M. Boudet de Paris have yet perceived the real nature or *modus operandi* of the remedy they adopted, or have recognized the value of "nerve vibration" in reference to any of the uses to which I have applied it besides the relief of pain.

I must crave the reader's indulgence for this digression. The question of priority in scientific work is, of course, of wholly subordinate importance, but it is a matter in which most investigators, who, like myself, have been deterred, by the fear of deceiving themselves and misleading others, from a hasty publication of "results," have need to take a modest interest.

It was not until long after the appearance of my last quoted paper that I was able to persuade myself that I should be justified in recommending the employment of mechanical vibration in the treatment of nerve states, other than those of which neuralgic pain was the urgent symptom.

On the 11th of March of the present year, the following paper appeared in the *British Medical Journal* :—

"PERCUSSION AS A THERAPEUTIC AGENT IN NERVOUS DISEASES.

"With the cognizance of the leading physiologists and neurologists in England and on the Continent, I have for some years past been employing carefully graduated and precisely applied percussion as a therapeutic agent in the treatment of nervous diseases and disturbances, on a principle of which the following statement, published by me in February, 1881, may be taken as a brief exposition. [I omit passages from *The Lancet*, sup. cit.]

"My method is, as will be seen from these extracts, based upon the hypotheses: (1) that all nerve action, whether normal or morbid, is vibratile; and (2) that it is possible to influence and control abnormal vibrations —in the manner above described—by mechanical vibrations propagated to the nervous structures, in *particular* directions and at *known* rates of speed. It is not my present purpose to discuss these hypotheses, or the method in detail; but I am anxious to re-state, and now affirm, certain propositions, founded on experience, which, in previous intimations of the progress and success of my experiments, I submitted tentatively. They are these—

"1. I have rarely failed, in a fairly large number of cases, many of them of several years' standing, to bring the cerebro-spinal and—sometimes directly at others in secondary circuits—the sympathetic ganglia, under control, by the application of my percuteur over, or in mechanical relation through the adjacent tissues with, those ganglia.

"2. I have in no instance failed to produce activity of the bowels, even in cases of previously obstinate constipation; and in many instances I have succeeded, within a short period, in restoring the periodic evacuation of their contents without recourse to drugs. This success alone places the method on a footing of value in daily practice.

"3. I can now, in result of my more recent experiments, propagate the vibrations I produce along the trunks and into the branches of most of the principal nerves, from their centres of origin, or call them into action, reflexly, through the afferent nerves connected with those centres. In limited paralyses, and even in circumscribed scleroses, this power is obviously of the highest therapeutic importance. Of course the like effect may be produced, and I admit, often more rapidly, with the electric current; but in the use of electricity we are projecting an external force into the organism, and one which always travels in the direction of least resistance; whereas the sole effect of vibration is to excite the centres and call out their potential energy, converting it into kinetic force. It can only act through the nerves.

"4. I can nearly always arouse torpid centres to action, and thus pave the way for their restoration to states of normal activity. Since it is physiologically certain that nutrition depends on exercise, and every part of the organism feeds in proportion as it works *healthily*, it is a great thing to be able to act thus directly on the nerve-centres which are the seats of energy.

"5. I can subdue the exaggerated reflex irritability of revolting subordinate centres, and replace them under control of the higher centres, even in cases of lateral sclerosis.

"Applying these facts—for such they undoubtedly are—to the needs of special nervous states, the practitioner will have no difficulty in perceiving that my method has great and obvious uses. I am anxious not to overstate the results I am obtaining, but they are such as to show that the physiological process of mechanical vibration is likely to prove a potent agent in the treatment of a wide range of maladies now most intractable. It will afford me much pleasure to show the process to any medical man who will call on me. It is impossible at present to describe its details in writing; but I will gladly aid any one in its application. My method has nothing in common with the "muscle-beating" and "shaking" recently introduced into this country; although my treatment was first tested in Paris. It is a system which must be approved and practised by the profession exclusively. Nothing do I so much dread as its falling into unprofessional hands. I have been engaged upon it since 1862, shortly after which date some of the first results were communicated to the Obstetrical Society of London."

In June last I had a paper in *The Lancet* (10th) giving the results of extended observations:—

"NERVE-VIBRATION AS A THERAPEUTIC AGENT.

"Enlarged experience in nerve vibration as a means or method of treating disease has confirmed my belief in its value, and I have no longer any hesitation in recommending its adoption by the profession. I do this with a full sense of the responsibility which necessarily attaches to the propounder of any strange doctrine in medicine, such as that which the theory of nerve vibration, undoubtedly, presupposes and implies ; and in an especial sense to the introducer of a new therapeutic agent. The responsibility of strongly urging a recourse to nerve-vibration, I am now fully prepared to accept. I commenced the investigation of nervous phenomena, first in connection with the various forms and causes of 'pain,' more than twenty years ago, and this method, which has been mentioned rather than recommended by me on several oceasions during the last few years, is the outcome of a long and careful series of experiments. I have now employed it in a very considerable number of cases, differing widely in their nature and characteristics, and although I have had many failures—mainly, as I believe, from errors in diagnosis and mismanagement in the application of the treatment—the net result has been such as to place beyond reasonable question the fact that in precisely applied mechanical vibration of nerves and nerve-centres, we have a means of eliciting function and stimulating nutrition which surpasses for directness and rapidity of action any other system or method extant. If this should seem to be an overstatement of the facts, it must be borne in mind that it is made in a medical journal, and with the knowledge that the profession will soon be able to verify or disprove the accuracy of my exertions.

"I do not propose to publish my cases immediately,

because sufficient time has not yet elapsed since the occurrence of what I conceive to have been 'cures' to show that they merited that description. At the same time, although as I have said, there are many obvious failures in my record of cases treated in this manner, the benefits which seem to have accrued from its adoption are so marked that I do not feel justified in longer delaying the step by which I place the means of forming a judgment on my method in the hands of the profession. Mr. Frederic Weiss, of the firm of Messrs. Weiss and Sons, has greatly aided me in producing, and will shortly be able to supply to members of the profession—I hope *exclusively*—a very satisfactory percuteur worked by electricity. I must acknowledge my indebtedness to Dr. George W. Balfour, of Edinburgh, for the recommendation to use electricity as a motive power. My deeply regretted friend the late Mr. Donald Napier advised me to employ this agent some five years ago, but I was then reluctant to do so lest it might be supposed that my process was in some way a modification of the use of electricity. It should, therefore, be understood that no current passes through the hammer of my instrument. The patient is not in the circuit. This force is, however, more convenient for sustained use than that obtained from the clock-spring in my mechanical percuteur. Messrs. Weiss and Sons have also a clock-work apparatus which has been made under my supervision, and which renders practicable what the French instruments have not, with a few exceptions, hitherto enabled me to accomplish. I will now briefly state the principles of the treatment, and leave it in the hands of the profession to give it a trial.

"In the treatment of neuralgia, I believe percussion acts simply by interrupting a morbid series of vibrations and substituting for it another series which is not morbid. Its success is by no means certain; but it deserves a trial, and particularly in cases which would otherwise be treated by nerve-stretching. When a nerve is stretched, it is, for a time at least, prevented from vibrating. When it is mechanically vibrated by percussion, it is compelled to fall into a new rhythm by the physical law of harmonies and discords, as explained in my first paper on this subject in *The Lancet*, February 19, 1881, p. 286. There are several modes of procedure. The percuteur may be applied over the seat of pain with varying force and speed until alleviation of the trouble is produced; or the percussion may be made higher up in the trunk of the nerve, over the centre, or at a more distant point in the periphery. If these methods fail, an attempt may be made to act upon the real or supposed seat of the pain indirectly through some other set of nerves. If success should not attend either of these modes of procedure, the irritation which causes the pain will probably be found to be reflected from some remote seat of disturbance, as in the case of pains in the heels from piles; and this seat of the exciting cause may generally be discovered by the physiological anatomist who will take the trouble to run over and exhaust the series of probabilities. The plan I suggest is, of course, far more exacting than the time-honoured expedient of giving an anodyne; but *relieving* and *curing* pain are two totally different processes, and it is only with the latter I have any concern.

"For the rousing of torpid nerve-centres and eliciting function from the several organs of the body, I believe nerve-vibration to be of the highest possible value. The recognised topography of the centres may serve as a rough guide for the application of the percuteur ; but as it is essential that the particular nerve energising the organ should be acted upon, and, as precisely as possible, that *only*, the operator will need to tax his knowledge of the nervous system in every case specifically. In a large proportion of instances the organ will have to be approached by a circuitous path, which can only be discovered by experiment in the individual case under treatment ; and the search for a way of reaching it must be made with a practical knowledge of the whole of its nervous connections. It should never be forgotten that the therapeutic agent is mechanical *nerve*-vibration ; and unless the nerve we want to stimulate is actually thrown into vibration it will not be excited to action. Every organ of the body, from the liver to the testicle, may, in the absence of utterly disabling organic disease, be made to perform its proper function by exciting the nerve, which supplies it with energy, by mechanical vibration. In this way I have seen the liver unloaded, and what seemed to be inveterate torpidity of the intestines, remedied in a few successive vibrations. I have now under treatment the case of a child who was six weeks ago to all appearance an idiot ; but who has already developed so much cerebral activity and growing intelligence under the influence of specific centre and nerve-vibration, that I entertain the strongest hope of his ultimate awakening, and a fair approach to the normal state. A surprising amount of success has attended percussion in cases of obstinate, and what was supposed to be irremediable, deafness. In a certain class of cases the hearing seems to have been recovered by arousing the auditory centre. In another class of instances of benefit derived I believe this has been due to the re-establishing of the mobility of the ossiculæ by mechanical vibration at a very high speed, the tonicity of the muscular fibres attached having been at the same time restored.

"In neurosthenia, neurasthenia, and even commencing sclerosis of the spinal cord with loss of tendon-reflex, the most remarkable effects are produced by applying the percuteur over the spinous processes of the appropriate vertebræ. I am afraid at present to publish some of the results recently gained. In a few cases I have wholly failed to do good, but in others—not a few—the "locomotor ataxy" has been removed or sensibly ameliorated, and the general improvement may be fairly described as astonishing. It is often necessary in this class of cases to combine proximate central percussion with lighter percussion at the remote periphery, especially when there is much trouble from lightning pains, or that creeping paralysis which so often first shows itself in the tibialis anticus. I believe Dr. Hughlings Jackson has somewhere noted this clinical fact, but, at the moment, I do not remember in what connection or where. In cases of exaggerated reflex irritability—a very common phenomenon, which is too generally overlooked or lightly regarded—I find the best plan of procedure to be by percussion over the seat of the irritability until that is removed, which generally happens after a very few applications of the percuteur. In a majority of my cases the subjugation of this irritable state has been almost immediately followed by motor improvement.

"In ordinary paralyses, which depend upon or are accompanied by deterioration of the muscles, I think nerve-vibration by percussion is inferior in value to electricity. In short, I do not think it has any appreciable effect except on the nerves themselves. It certainly improves the nutrition of nervous tissue, and this indirectly promotes the nutrition of muscles, but the process is circuitous and slow. Faradaism is a preferable remedy. Nerve vibration is not the rival of electricity. The two agents act in totally different manners. Vibration simply excites a nerve centre to such activity as it may have strength or power to perform. It does not impart any new energy or introduce any new force to the system. Electricity infuses an extraneous force into the organism, but with this drawback, that it is impossible to ensure its acting only on the nerve it is desired to stimulate, and solely in such a way as to render any act of that nerve *its own*, and therefore normal. Vibration cannot possibly act in any other way than through the nerve or upon the centre, and, in a strict sense, nervously. One curious effect of percussion may be more interesting to the physiologist than to the practitioner, but I will place it on record. Playing over the centre from which the nerves supplying a particular set of muscles arise is apt to produce a feeling of fatigue or stiffness which may seem to be located in the leg or arm, although the extremity itself is not touched. This will help to explain how what is called nightmare may produce cramp, and how the activity of certain automatic centres in a wearying dream of action may give rise to a sense of fatigue on waking.

"These few hints will serve to point the practitioner to a method of procedure in making trial of the remedy, but all I know of the method is at the disposal of any member of the profession who may desire to be more fully or precisely informed. I will only say, in conclusion, that I am very hopeful that nerve vibration will enable us to cure maladies which have hitherto been beyond remedy; and that in a certain class of cases—namely, those which require the direct stimulation of nerve-centres for their recovery—this agent will greatly help, perhaps supersede, the use of drugs."

This, I fear, somewhat too egotistical summary of the history of the investigations in which I have been engaged, and of the communications which have from time to time been made to the profession with a view to bring the subject under its notice, clears the way for a brief review of the principles of nerve vibration and excitation in the treatment of functional and organic disease, as I now understand and interpret the facts I have been able to collate, and the system of physiological treatment which they have suggested.

THE PRINCIPLE.

GENERAL OUTLINE OF THE TREATMENT AND DESCRIPTION OF THE APPARATUS.

It is necessary at the outset to distinguish between *vibration* and *excitation*. The former does not always, though it does generally, involve or induce the latter; and the latter, that is, excitation of a nerve, may probably be effected by other means than vibration, even when a vibratile body or instrument is employed to excite the nerve, and although the nerve is undoubtedly thrown into a state of vibration as soon as it becomes excited. The explanation of this seeming paradox may be attempted as follows:—When the practical physiologist—(the only interrogator of Nature, whose results are wholly worthy and entirely trustworthy, I mean the vivisectionist)—draws his needle with a light hand across the sheath of a nerve, or presses the point of his instrument upon it steadily, he excites the nerve or centre, which means that he throws it into vibration. The reader who is familiar with Dr. Sydney Ringer's beautiful exposition of the action of blisters, in his classical work on Therapeutics, will not need to be reminded that blisters, mustard poultices, and certain other remedies, which may be classed as specific irritants, act in this way, namely, by throwing nervous tissue—I mean nerve fibres and cells—into particular formulæ of vibration. Some produce large and slow waves, others small and quick vibratile movements, with characteristic effects. A knowledge of this fact lies at the root of the comprehension of the difference between vibration and excitation. A nerve may, as I have said, be excited without being directly vibrated by the excitor, which may not, perhaps, be itself perceptibly vibrating, although the excitement produced is vibratile. And the physical effect of a vibrating instrument may be to excite by irritating, as the needle point of the biological experimenter excites, instead of inducing nerve action by directly propagating its own vibration to the nervous tissue.

I say the recognition of this difference of method in producing the desired result, namely, nerve action, must be made at the outset, because it is essential to a scientific use of the new remedy which I propose for adoption that there should be no mistake as to its *modus operandi* in each particular case or form of administration. I have myself seen reason to modify my first notion of the treatment in this respect. When I commenced my experiments with the percuteur I thought that, in every instance, the effect produced was due to the propagation of the vibration set up in, or by, the instrument to the nerve on which I was operating. I now believe, that in some instances, the effect is rather due to the excitation of the nerve by the first two or three blows of the hammer. The practical inference I have been led to draw from the recognition of this fact —and I expect other investigators will be driven to the same conclusion—is that it is desirable to use the percuteur very delicately at first, particularly in cases of neuralgia, and to touch the skin over the painfully vibrating nerve sheaths lightly and quickly, rather than to keep it playing on the part, as was at first my practice. I mention this matter in this connection, because, although it relates to the practice rather than the principle of the treatment, it throws strong illustrative light on the distinction I am seeking to enforce between vibration and excitation.

In starting from the physiological stand-point, as regards nerve action, which I have incidentally taken up in the introductory observations, it will be obvious that the aim of the therapeutist who employs vibration must be to throw the nerve into a *new* state of activity. This is equally true, whether he be trying to rouse a torpid centre or to change the rhythm of a morbid state. My notion of morbid activity is this. I believe, as previously affirmed, that under normal conditions, when a nerve cell or fibre becomes active, the one in receiving impressions or discharging force, the other in transmitting sensory impressions or reflex or direct motor impulses, the essential elements of the nervous tissue vibrate mechanically in their beds or cylinders. When either the vibrations of cell or nerve are unrhythmical in themselves or discordant with the vibrations of other cells or nerves, which they may either throw into disorder or inhibit (perhaps this is the true explanation of the "inhibitory" process), they propagate the commotion the disturbance has set up to their sheaths or envelopes, and the activity becomes disorderly and painful.

I carry this hypothesis so far that my theory of a cold, for example, as I have stated it, for the laity, elsewhere, is as follows:—

"When the surface of the body or the air-passages are chilled by a draught, or by being drenched with rain and sitting in cold damp clothes, lying in damp sheets, and the like, the mischievous impression is made, not on the skin itself or on the lining membrane of the air-passages, but upon the vast net-work of minute nerve-filaments which lie beneath these membranes, and connect the surfaces of the body—both external and internal—with the nerve-centres, which are the sources and *foci* of energy and power. These nerve-centres receive, through the multitudinous branches of telegraph-like nerves, a shock or staggering impression that for the moment paralyses them; and, so long as this paralysis or stupefaction lasts, another part of the nervous system, called the vaso-motor, or vessel-contracting centre, whose peculiar function it is to regulate the calibre of the blood-vessels, gets the upper hand, and these blood-vessels are contracted so that they carry less blood than usual, the smaller branches of the arterial system which form a net-work immediately underneath the skin and give it its bright pink colour are so reduced in 'bore' or calibre—as an elastic or compressible tube may be reduced—that the red blood does now flow through them, and the surface looks pallid. Presently comes the recovery from this state, or the 'reaction,' as it is called, when the first effects of the shock have passed off and the centres revive. Now occurs the critical moment. If the torpor has been great, and the recovery is slow or imperfect, as often happens in a depressed or what is called 'delicate' state of the organism, the vaso-motor centre, which of course shares the general weakness, will give way before the reaction is established ; and then the heart, pumping its blood into yielding and unstrung vessels, dilates them, and local congestions or accumulations of blood may take place ; while the absence of proper resistance excites the heart to tumultuous action, and the disturbances of fever and inflammation occur. It is a question of balance in power between two parts of the nervous system, the general and the particular—the latter being, as I have said, the centre which regulates the calibre of the blood-vessels—and this practically resolves itself into a question of time. If the reaction of the general nervous system is quick, there is a rush of blood to the surface vessels, and, due resistance being found, the heart quickens its pump-like action, and the sweat-glands are thrown into activity, so that perspiration ensues .If, on the other hand, the vaso-motor centre has participated in the shock, the blood propelled to the surface simply dilates the vessels, and the skin remains dry ; there is rapid action of the heart because there is an obstacle to overcome, but the current of the blood moves slowly. Coincident with these purely physical actions and reactions, involving a departure from the healthy condition of matter as regards the function of the nerve-centres and the circulation of the blood, are disturbances of the chemical processes of health and consequently alteration in the nutritive relation of the tissues of the body and the blood ; but these changes are too complicated to be discussed in this article, and it is not important to the solution of the question before us that they should be immediately considered. What then is 'a cold?' I reply, it is a disturbance of the balance between the several parts of the nervous system, brought about by the shock of a sudden or prolonged exposure to the depressing effects of chill ; but the same physico-vital results may be produced in the organism by the operation of any agent which is capable of giving the nervous system a similar shock and creating the same kind of disturbance."

This may appear a digression, but its bearing on the question under discussion will be apparent when I add that, in my judgment, "Nature's provisions against 'a cold,' in so far as that may be the effect of a chill, are two—sneezing and shivering. A violent fit of sneezing often saves a chilled body the consequences of a depressing influence. The nerve centres are aroused, the heart's action is stimulated, and the blood is thrown to the surface by the convulsive and explosive action. If sneezing fails, or sometimes in its absence if the chill be great and deep, an intense and prolonged fit of shivering may arouse the latent and, as it were, suddenly-suppressed forces of the nervous system. It, however, commonly happens that, when the chill is so intense as to produce deep shivering, the mischief done is too serious to admit of a prompt reaction. Thus it comes to pass that the common saying is true : sneezing shows that the cold will be slight, while shivering, and particularly only a very brief but deep shiver, portends a severe congestion or inflammation in some organ. When organic blood and other poisons act on the nerve-centres, shivering is a very bad sign, as a rule. In cases of threatened cold from chill, sneezing, and occasionally shivering, produce perspiration. When this occurs, and the sweating is profuse, with a warm and reddened surface, the 'cold' is likely to be prevented. It is not the perspiration that does the good, but the outbreak of a hot sweat shows that the arteries are offering healthy resistance to the current of the blood; and it is then probable that the balance of force between the heart and the vessels will be quickly re-established in such manner that the functions of the circulation may be duly performed and disturbances which would otherwise end in disease may be prevented."

Dr. Hugh Campbell, who has for some time past been employing nerve-vibration, has published the following particulars in *The British Medical Journal.* They aptly illustrate the view just taken; and show its direct bearing on the question under discussion. He writes:—

"In a case which I was recently treating by nerve-vibration, the patient presented himself one day with all the indications of a sharp attack of influenza—injected conjunctivæ, frontal headache, &c. Percussion over the superior cervical ganglia, within a few minutes, unexpectedly removed both the objective and subjective symptoms."

To return; the aim of the vibration treatment is, I say, to throw the nervous tissue into a *new* state or series of vibrations. There are, therefore, two parts or stages of its action: first, that of change, either from quiescence to motion, or from one form of action to another; and second the establishment of a new activity. The first part relates to rousing, the second to continuing vibratile activity of the nerve elements. It is in relation to the action of the percuteur in "arousing" that the recognition of the difference which I have already pointed out, between the two modes of its action, is chiefly important. If a nerve or nerve centre is in itself healthy, though dormant, it will suffice to awake it; and percussion is simply useful as a convenient and precise mode of effecting this limited purpose. Any other would do as well, if it could be as directly applied, and as effectually restrained from setting up collateral vibrations which may prove injurious or render the first feeble efforts of the nerve or centre to act nugatory by interference. In my experience of the percussion, small as it has yet been, I have known one or two touches with the percuteur rouse a nerve, and call it into permanent action. A curious instance of this occurred to me recently. A patient under treatment by vibration for dyspepsia dependent on inactivity of the fibres of the muscular coat of the stomach, was, I found, suffering from an injury to the spermatic cord, which seemed to have produced paralysis of the cremaster. The testicle of the affected side had dropped to such an extent that a suspensory bandage required to be continually worn, and caused great inconvenience. I applied the percuteur for a few moments over the inguinal branch of the genito-crural nerve, with the effect of very quickly producing contraction of the cremaster. After one or two applications, the patient left off his bandage, and has never suffered from the trouble since. In this instance, the action of the percuteur had, obviously, only been of a rousing nature; and it simply had the effect of awakening a torpid nerve from the prolonged slumber into which it had been thrown by an injury. This will sufficiently explain what I have called the first stage or form of the action of vibration. It is needless to recal to the recollection of the reader how a blow on the head will sometimes rouse the inert cells of the cerebrum, with the result of converting a stupid brain into one of at least average intellectual ability.

The first effect of nerve-vibration, therefore, is awakening or interrupting; the second is more like tuning a violin string, or the wire of a pianoforte. Nerve-stretching acts in one of two ways for a time. If much force be used it disorganizes the nerve and prevents *any* vibration taking place in its elements, with the result, in successful cases, of giving it a new starting-point when the integrity of the nerve-fibre is restored in the process of natural repair. When less force is used, the nerve is acted upon precisely as screwing and stretching act on a violin string, altering its physical capacity for vibration, and either reducing or increasing the amplitude of the waves of movement into which agitation will throw it. I doubt not that nerves of different calibres have each their proper physical capacities for vibration; and the vibrations of a nerve are, in perfect health, mathematically component and complementary parts of the vibrations of the trunk from which it springs. When a nerve becomes turgid from congestion, or is in any way swollen or attenuated, this perfect relation is disturbed, and the result is functional disorder, and probably pain.

The manner in which vibration acts in the second stage or phase of its process is, I believe, explained by the law of musical concords and discords or harmonies. We interrupt by a discord, and control by substituting one set of vibrations for another. In this way, by vibrating a particular nerve daily, as nearly as possible at the same hour and for the same length of time, with a percuteur working at the same speed or number of vibrations per second, we may educate the nerve-cells or fibres, so to say, to a new rhythmical habit, and thus establish new vibratile conditions. It is of the highest moment to recognize this fact. We may not at first be able to ascertain the precise rate or rhythm of normal nerve vibrations—which I believe to bear a definite proportional relation to the size of the nerve—this will come to our knowledge later on ; but meanwhile we can change the state and establish new conditions, and although the feat is performed in the dark and clumsily, the result to the patient is often singularly successful. We have lifted him out of the painful or morbid state, although what that was, and how his amended state differs from the old one, we are not yet able to ascertain.

The reader will gather from this crude and confessedly clumsy statement of my views how I believe nerve-vibration acts. I adopt percussion as a mode of throwing the nerve fibres and cells into vibration, simply because it seems the readiest and the most manageable; but if it should be hereafter superseded by some better mode of effecting vibration, I shall be the first to hail the improvement as a further development of the method of treatment in which I am interested, and which I beg the profession to study and test. In practice it will be found that the number of blows given by the percuteur must be varied, if we are to attain our object. As a rule it is better to attack a large nerve, or a dull, grinding pain, or a "numbness," with a high rate of small vibrations; and a small peripheral nerve, or a very acute "fine," needle-like pain, with comparatively slow and large vibrations. In the difference we are most likely to secure discord to interrupt, or induce a change of state. If we could only ascertain precisely the rate or character of the morbid vibrations, we could, of course, by the law of musical concords, at once apply the remedy in an appropriate form. The point to remember, is that it is with the nerve we have to deal, not with its surroundings; but these surroundings which lie between us and the nerve on which we wish to operate require careful consideration. It is useless vibrating over a nerve or centre unless we can reach it. As a rule, the mere position of a nerve or centre in topographical relation to the surface of the body is not of the first importance; sometimes it is possible to act on a centre through the adjacent bones. Often, for example, though not always, the spinal cord may be vibrated by playing on the spinous processes of the vertebræ. In this way I can occasionally send an impulse along a particular nerve, but the experiment is by no means uniformly successful.

In the majority of instances it fails. As a rule it is better to try to act on the centre, along the physiological line of communication—namely, the afferent nerve. In cases of "locomotor ataxy," and in some other morbid states, reflex movements may be readily called forth by operating upon the cutaneous nerves or over large mixed nerves, such as the anterior tibial.

It will be understood that in no instance, and under no circumstance, can the mere agitation of a purely efferent or motor nerve produce muscular contraction. No "force" is communicated by the hammer of the percuteur. It simply vibrates the nerve elements, and any movement produced must be due to the calling out of nerve force from the centre. In short, the vibration must be projected along the afferent fibres to the centre, where activity of the cells is excited, with the result of provoking a discharge of nervous force—whatever that may be—along the efferent nerve to the muscle which contracts. It is scarcely possible to call out force by this process of vibration in a healthy subject. Occasionally a very little action is produced in individual cases, particularly when the percuteur is applied over tendons at the precise point of their connection with muscular fibres, but never, so far as I can detect, at any other point. When, however, there is either torpidity or an excess of irritability, owing to the existence of some block in the motor line of communication, vibration of the afferent nerve seems to incite the centre to discharge its pent up force. I have utilized this effect to obviate a tendency to spasm, by exhausting the motor force of certain centres in the spinal cord, with the effect of reducing that "irritability" which I believe to be the main cause of the difficulty in walking in locomotor ataxy, a difficulty wholly distinct from the loss of sensation, which is due to affections of the posterior columns of the cord. Perhaps the most curious and suggestive results have, in my experience, been found in cases of lateral sclerosis. When the limbs jerk and fly off at tangents in trying to do anything, this is clearly not because there is loss of sensation, since it is equally apparent before and after the foot touches the ground, or the hand comes into contact with any object! The motor force discharged by the action of the cerebral centres upon the automatic centres is unable to travel along the proper nerve, and goes off in the direction of least resistance. We call this "inco-ordination," but that term only designates the phenomenon without in any degree explaining its nature or discovering its cause, which I believe to be that above mentioned. When the irritability of the centre has been exhausted reflexly by vibration of the nerves in connection with it, there is generally, for a time at least, marked increase in the power, or possibility, of voluntary motion and co-ordination. One interesting fact in relation to the process of excitation by nerve-vibration may be mentioned here. All the movements excited by percussion of the nerves in a limb have a tendency to be repeated. I have frequently incited a centre to perform a particular series of automatic movements as many as four or five times in succession, with intervals of ten or fifteen seconds, by a few minutes' vibration with the percuteur, the movements being repeated while I sat by and watched. Sometimes the observer notices the contraction of the muscles before the patient is aware of what his limbs are doing ; at others he will tell the operator that they are "going to do something" before the latter can detect any movement. I should here explain that, with a view to eliminate possible sources of error in the study of these phenomena, I have never yet percussed a female patient, and have not founded any of my conclusions on the treatment of hysterical males. This is a matter of much moment in my judgment, and I am, therefore, careful to place the fact on record. I have avoided, and shall continue to avoid, the treatment of women by percussion, simply because I do not want to be hoodwinked, and help to mislead others, by the vagaries of the hysterical state or the characteristic phenomena of mimetic disease.

Enough has been said to indicate the outlines of the principle ; I now turn to the apparatus. At first I used

FIG. I.

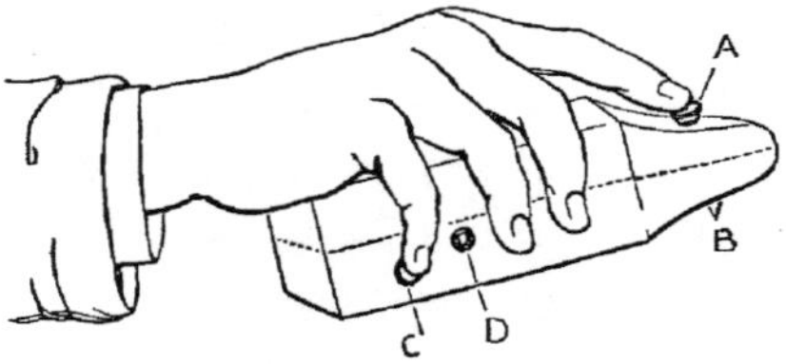

The Clockwork Percuteur, showing the mode of using it.

D, winding-up pivot. C, ivory button ; while this is pressed by the finger, the hammer continues in action ; when the pressure is taken off it stops. A. By pressing this button the length of stroke can be increased, and the speed slightly reduced, while the force of the blow is augmented. B, the pointed ivory hammer with which the percussion is made. A flat-headed hammer, or brush, can be substituted for the ivory point.

clockwork percuteurs, and some of the most notable results I have gained in practice have been obtained with these instruments ; but, except for the treatment of neuralgia—and in bad cases of that intractable malady—I do not recommend these instruments. The

FIG. 2.

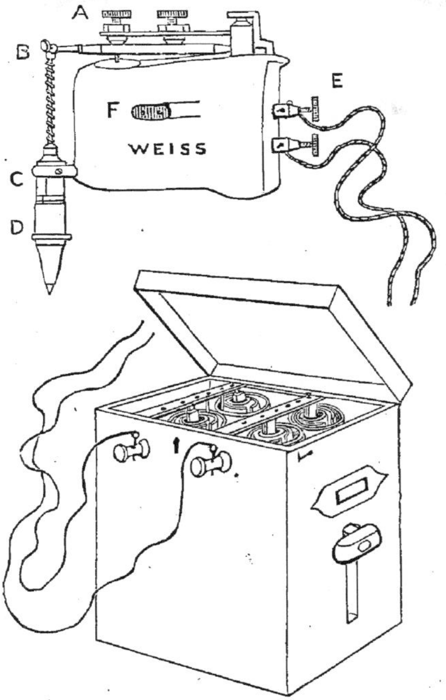

The Percuteur worked by electro-magnetism, and the *Bunsen's Battery*, as supplied by Messrs. Weiss & Sons.

(I am indebted to the late Mr. Donald Napier and Dr. George W. Balfour, of Edinburgh, for the suggestion to use electricity as a motive power for the percuteur.)

E, screws connecting battery wires with the percuteur. A, screws for making connection. There are two; either may be used. That neares the hinge of the vibrator causes the hammer to beat at the highest speed. B, screw for attaching the hammer, brushes, &c., to the instrument. C, brass cylinder through which the rod of the hammer passes. D, vulcanite tube, which is attached with a screw, and regulates the length of the stroke made by the hammer. F, button which, being pressed or pushed with the finger, sets the percuteur going.

percuteur worked by electricity is, in every way, superior to the clockwork instrument, except as regards portability. In consulting-room practice, the electric instrument answers every purpose most efficiently. The general practitioner will, however, need to provide himself with the clockwork percuteur for use at his patient's house; and, as I have said, although seemingly very weak in its blow, and troublesome, because it requires

FIG. 3.

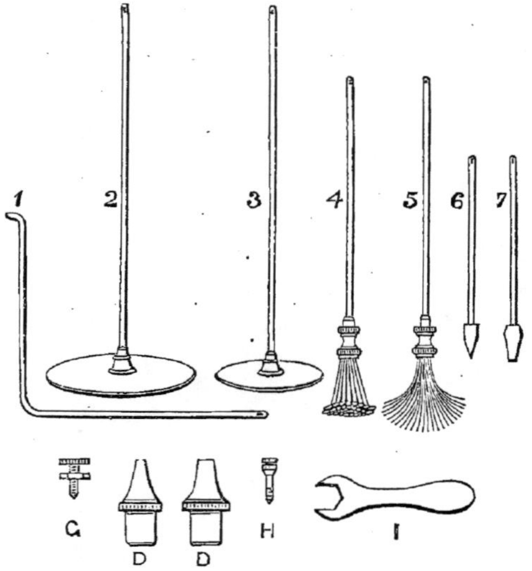

7, Flat-headed hammer; 6, pointed hammer; 5, light brush for relief of superficial pain and to redden the surface; 4, hard brush. This brush grew out of a suggestion made by Dr. Hugh Campbell, and is very effective; 3, small disc; 2, large disc for use in water; 1, bent hammer. G, connection screw, tipped with platinum; D, D, vulcanite tubes to protect hammers; H, screw to attach hammer to percuteur; I, clamp to fix connecting screws.

to be frequently wound, it is by no means ineffectual. The above diagrams will show the instruments and their adjuncts. What little I have to say of their use may be said most conveniently in the course of the detailed observations I propose to make on nerve-vibration in practice.

NERVE-VIBRATION AND EXCITATION IN PRACTICE.

FOR THE RELIEF OF PAIN.

If I am right in my theory that pain occurs when vibrations of the essential elements of nervous tissue extend to the beds of cells and the sheaths of nerve fibres, it is easy to understand how compression of a nerve,—either by force applied directly to its trunk, as when the ulnar nerve is squeezed as it passes behind the inner condyle of the humerus, or by distension of the surrounding tissues from congestion of the vessels, or by effusion—causes pain, and why the pain is proportioned to the constriction, short of extreme pressure, which must, of course, altogether prevent vibration of the nerve affected. As the nerve is compressed, its sheath is forced in upon the nerve elements, and necessarily becomes irritated by their disorderly vibrations. Without such an explanation as this theory of pain affords, it has always seemed to me unaccountable, that so little pressure—a very little at the most—as can be caused by the congestion of a swollen finger, should occasion so much agony as is experienced, for example, in whitlow; or that the throbbing of the arteries, should be as acutely and painfully felt as we know to be the fact. In this way also one branch of a nerve whose sheath is vibrating painfully, may communicate its vibration to another sheath which happens to be in juxtaposition. In the treatment of pain by vibration, it is necessary to determine, as precisely as possible, the particular branch in which it is located, and to act, in the first instance at least, upon that alone. The treatment will fail if healthy or normally vibrating nerves are mechanically vibrated with those which are in a morbid state. It is, accordingly, important to localize the seat of the disturbance in pain, and to apply the percuteur as directly as may be, to the disorderly and disturbing branch alone.

The *rationale* of the process of relief is to overpower the tumultuous vibration of the nerve elements within their sheath, by communicating an independent and different vibratile motion to the nerve as a whole. In the attempt to do this, the pain is for the moment frequently increased ; but this exacerbation of the distressed sensation, which is the contingent consequence of an augmented tumult, rapidly subsides—if it occurs, which is not always the case—as soon as the elements are compelled to fall into the same rhythmical vibration as that communicated to their sheath by the regular beat of the percuteur; the discord between the nerve elements and their sheath, which is the cause of the pain, and the sensation subsiding together. If the mechanical vibration, communicated to the nerve by percussion, fail to overpower the morbid vibration of the nerve elements, it is likely to aggravate the suffering. When, therefore, the pain of neuralgia is not quickly relieved by vibration, it is wrong to continue it with the same instrument working at the same speed.

The mechanical percuteurs (Fig. 1, page 57) are provided with a pressure movement (A, Fig. 1, page 57) which lengthens the stroke of the hammer, and thus diminishes its speed, while increasing its force at pleasure, and the electrical percuteurs (Fig. 2, page 58) have two contact pins (A, Fig. 2, page 58) one at the extremity, and the other half-way along the length of the vibrator, which respectively give different rates of vibration. If the pain does not pass away almost immediately after a momentary increase, to which I have previously alluded as being often produced by the first agitation of the nerve sheath, in short, within a few seconds of the application of the percuteur, it is well to change the rate of the percussion. Another point of moment is to withdraw the percuteur instantly when the pain is relieved, and wait until it returns, which it is almost sure to do in a few minutes. Then touch it again. I find that the pain returns sometimes with increased acuteness, if the percussion has been rapid—as many as three or four times in as many minutes—before it finally ceases. The application should be precise and very light, and it ought to cease the very moment the pain ceases. By continuing the vibration too long—that is, after relief has been obtained—a new vibration, equally disorderly and painful with that we are trying to relieve, may be set up by the percussion. Great care and tact are necessary in treating pain by nerve-vibration. The aim should always be to gain the desired result with the least force of blow, and the shortest duration of percussion, restricted within the smallest practicable area. By mismanagement failure may be secured and the treatment discredited. For some months after I commenced my experiments, I was unsuccessful in the majority of instances, and I began to doubt the value of the remedy; but, since arriving at the general rules for percussion which I have now tried to make plain, I have seldom failed, at least with the electrical percuteur. The mechanical instrument is very uncertain in its effects, even in the improved form in which it is now offered to the profession. The French instruments, which I tried to use two years ago, must, I fear, looking to the very small proportion of instances in which they prove efficient for the purpose of relieving pain, be pronounced failures.

The relief of pain, though by no means the most important, is undoubtedly one of the most urgent and widely persistent claims which humanity makes on the physician and his art, and it was in the search for an efficient and rational mode of treating this grievous symptom or concomitant of disease, I came to perceive the nature of pain, and first made the attempt to allay it as one would put an end to discord in the vibration of a musical reed instrument. My interest in the success of the method in this particular sphere of its action is, therefore, exceedingly great, and I would venture to ask and urge all who may try the treatment to give the subject their special attention. I can only repeat what I said in my first paper in *The Lancet*, namely, that I attribute my failures to faults in the method of applying the instrument. One of my earliest and commonest blunders was to press too heavily on the part affected. I now find that the slightest touch with the point of the hammer is incomparably more successful. At first I vibrated the whole of the surrounding tissues, and especially the adjacent bones. For example, to relieve neuralgic pain in the branches of the fifth, I percussed strongly either over the superior margin of the orbit at or near the exit of the supra-orbital branch, or upon the superior maxilla or malar bone for the infra-orbital branch, or on the lower jaw at or near the emergence of the mental branch for pain in the inferior division of the fifth. I failed as often as I succeeded. Now I try to hit on the exact point to which the pain is referred, if it be superficial, or to find some terminal twig in close anatomical relation with the deep branch which is vibrating painfully, and with the least possible pressure of the pointed hammer (No. 6, Fig. 3, page 59) I percuss very rapidly, if the pain be of a dull grinding character, or at a lower speed if the pain be exceedingly sharp, and move the instrument slowly over the skin until it touches the precise spot at which the pain is located when, for the moment perhaps, it is increased, but very quickly afterwards relieved. This I take to be the principle of the treatment for the relief of pain. If the pain cannot be localized, but seems to extend over a considerable area, the operator may use the disc (No. 3, Fig. 3, page 59) very lightly, applying it to the surface ; or in cases of extreme tenderness, for example, if the pain be situated in an inflamed limb or joint, he may immerse the foot in water, about the temperature of the skin over the seat of the suffering, and vibrate through the water, holding the disc in the fluid, and passing it round the painful part, about an inch

FIG. 4.

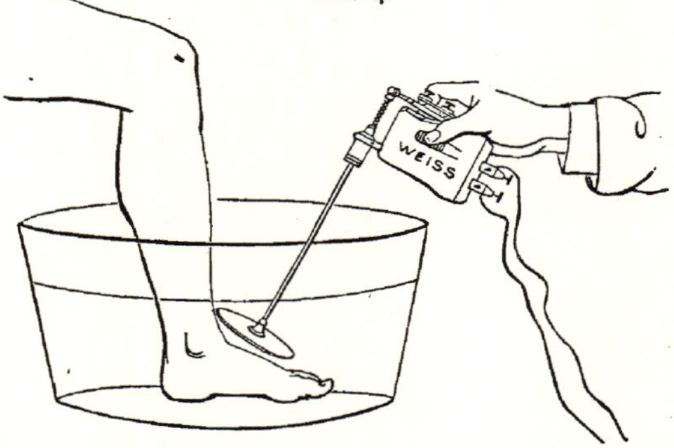

from its surface, without touching it. The sketch will show the mode of using the disc in the manner described.

FIG. 5.

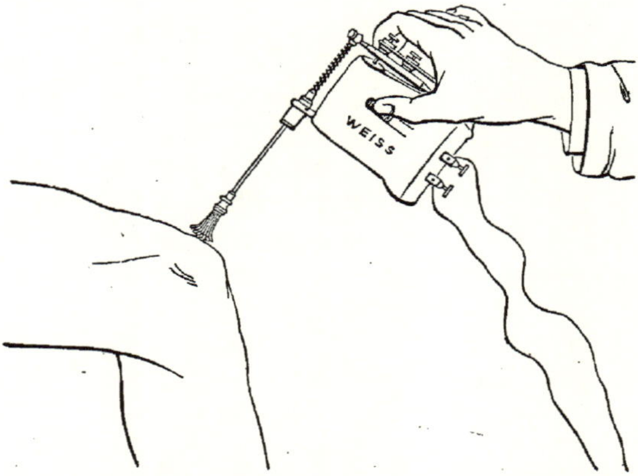

In other cases, when the pain is either entirely superficial, perhaps of a formicating, or tingling, or burning character, or when it seems to be deeply seated below a dull and morbid skin—two apparently opposite conditions—it is well to use one of the wire brushes (Nos. 4, 5, Fig. 3, p. 59), as shown in Fig. 5 (p. 65), passing it lightly over the surface; or in some forms of deep-seated pain, pressing it firmly on the skin.

The practitioner will discover the best plan of proceeding very readily after a few experiments, and he will recognize the difficulty of giving precise directions for treatment. No two cases, though closely similar, are identical in their requirements, and the treatment must differ

FIG. 6.

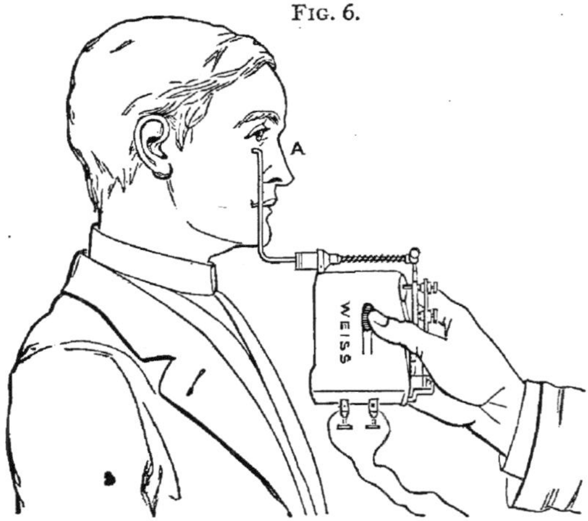

with the state. For the relief of pain in many regions, the bent rod hammer (No. 1, Fig. 3, p. 59), will be found exceedingly useful, applied as above (Fig. 6). It can be brought to bear on almost any nerve which lies fairly near the surface. When the nerve affected is wholly out of reach, relief is often obtained by vibrating some afferent branch, which proceeds to the same, or an adjacent centre, or which passes near the trunk of the affected nerve in some part of its course. Cases of headache are generally best treated by percussion with the disc over the meatus of the ear, or with the flat-headed hammer (No. 7, Fig. 3, p. 59) over the superior cervical nerves and plexuses. Parietal headache may often be relieved by percussion over the transverse root of the zygoma; and occipital by percussion about an inch behind the posterior margin of the base of the mastoid process, on the superior curved ridge of the occipital bone, or the percuteur may be moved slowly along the ridge two or three times. For this last purpose it is well to use the pointed ivory hammer. Hemicranial headache is best treated with the brush, applied very lightly to the scalp, and moved from below upwards and from before backwards, a few times in an orderly manner. The patient should, in all cases of percussion for pain, be told to speak the moment relief, however slight it may be, is perceived, and the operator should instantly suspend the percussion until the pain returns, or if it has not quite subsided, increases. A series of experiments with the percuteur used for the purpose in the manner described, will give the practitioner a better knowledge of its powers and defects than could be conveyed by many pages of description.

For the Control of Disorderly Movements.

Choreic movements are generally due to an excess of irritability in some centre, which renders it ever ready to discharge its nervous force on the slightest excitation, or even without the application of any provocation from without. Convulsive movements and twitches—tricks as they are called—are generally worse when the nervous system as a whole is excited, and particularly when the higher centres—the organs of consciousness—are specially active. There is what Dr. Hughlings Jackson has significantly designated a barrel-organ arrangement, which favours the repetition of combined or formulated movements whenever the centres become surcharged as it were, by the accumulation of nervous force. What has been done once will be done again, because the first act has left the molecules of the automatic centres as a train ready to carry the explosive force a second time along the same nerves, and so on until the barrel organ, whenever it acts at all, plays the same tune. Nerve vibration by percussion is decidedly useful in these cases. The method of applying it may be briefly described as follows :—Strive to impress the centres by percussing mixed or afferent nerves on that side or surface of the limb which is opposite to the line or direction of the choreic movement, or by percussing nerves through which antagonistic muscles might—if the case were a suitable one—be called into action reflexly. For example, if the flexors and pronators of the arm contract convulsively, percuss the nerves most likely to act reflexly on the extensors and supinators. To do any real good the percuteur must, in cases of this class, be played strongly with considerable motive force—using, say, eight cells of the Bunsen battery—and employing either the flat-headed hammer or the hard brush. If the latter be employed, it must be held firmly but not pressed on the skin, the object being to secure the heaviest practicable blow, which is best secured by holding it so that the points of the wires rise clear of the skin each time the current is broken, in order to take advantage of the full momentum of the impact when the blow is struck. The percuteur may be made to trace the principal nerves upwards, and the percussion kept up for fully twenty minutes daily. If the face is habitually contorted, percuss the nerves which carry sensation from the skin covering the opposing muscles. For example, if the zygomatic muscles are in the habit of twitching with the orbicularis palpebrarum, percuss a little above the eyebrow; and around the mouth over the orbicularis, and the triangularis, oris specially. In cases of general chorea, percussion down the spine, while the patient sits across a chair or on a stool, is serviceable. The flat-headed hammer should be used with a good deal of force, and the aim should be to vibrate the roots of the spinal nerves, percussing as nearly as possible over the interspaces of the transverse processes. The percuteur should be passed down the back close on either side of the spinous processes, resting a few moments at each, and persisting wherever pain is produced by the percussion, *until* it subsides. There is often considerable irritability of the posterior branches of the nerves in these cases, and not uncommonly neuralgic tenderness over the vertebræ. These local symptoms are speedily relieved by the vibration, and as the cure succeeds in this particular, the choreic movements are at first less strong, and then less frequent, until they gradually disappear. The seventh cervical vertebræ should always be vibrated for flying "twitches," and it is well in cases of this class to explore the whole length of the spine, with a view to discover any local excitability or "tenderness." I have not had any large experience in these cases, but what I have seen of the effects of nerve-vibration in chorea, gives me great hope of its usefulness. If it should answer as well as I anticipate, it will prove a boon to the family practitioner, who is often consulted for the remedy of "tricks" and "grimaces" of the young. If these are neglected, or not cured in youth, they often become confirmed and very troublesome later on in life.

TO ELICIT ENERGY FROM TORPID CENTRES.

When the symptoms of disease, or the absence of some function, point to the torpidity of a special nerve centre, it is necessary to approach it by the physiological rather than the anatomical route, although in a large proportion of instances the two are identical. The afferent nerves offer the best, and often the only practicable line of communication. For example, if there be failure, or absence, of sexual power, the state may often be remedied by percussing with the pointed percuteur over the inguinal nerves and those of the perineum, rather than by percussion with the flat-headed hammer over the second lumbar vertebræ, which would seem to be the most likely mode of procedure—with a view to vibrate the genito-urinary centre by strong percussion through the spine. Cases of this defect or deficiency differ greatly. I have frequently failed to do any good by percussing the spine, but certainly failure is rare when the centre is approached reflexly. I believe it is possible to act on any centre with the effect of sensibly improving its nutrition by vibrating its afferent nerves. The cerebral centres are best reached by percussing with the disc applied over the ear, or with the flat-headed hammer at the root of the zygomatic process of the temporal bone, immediately in front of the auditory meatus, also at the external angular process of the frontal bone, and along the superior curved line of the occipital bone. The centres of special sense are to be approached through their terminal organs. The optic, by very gentle vibration of the globe of the eye through the closed lid, a florin being used as a shield, and the flat-headed hammer being lightly applied; or the small disc (No. 3, Fig. 3, p. 59), may be used if the eye be not too sunken. The olfactory centres may be stimulated by vibration of the vertical plate of the ethmoid bone with the pointed hammer, applied exactly on the median line at the root of the nose ; or with the bent arm hammer passed into the nose and allowed to play gently upwards and inwards on the cribriform plates. This operation, needs, of course, to be performed very carefully with a light hand, and considerable judgment. The gustatory centres may be roused, and taste restored in many cases, by percussing the mucous membrane of the tongue with the bent arm hammer or the small disc, or the brush held sideways so as to vibrate the papilla laterally with the everted tips of its outer edge, the tongue being protruded, and lying on the lower teeth. The point to bear in mind is that even when it seems easy to act directly on a centre, it is better to try to rouse it through its afferent nerves. No *immediate* effect, is, of course, to be anticipated in cases of this class, but by persevering percussion, most centres may be aroused, their nutrition improved, and their energy of function elicited.

To Allay Morbid Irritability.

This is, in my judgment, one of the most interesting—from a scientific point of view—of the many purposes nerve-vibration can be employed to effect. The operation may be studied to great advantage in the treatment of locomotor ataxy. In the course of the disease or diseases—for I believe there are several—which have loss of " co-ordination" for one of their prominent symptoms, it will soon be apparent to the careful clinical observer that the essential morbid condition is a block or undue resistance in the course of the motor nerves. The notion that loss of sensation, is the primary fault, may be dissipated by a simple familiar experiment. Tell an ataxic patient to place his toe on a particular spot of the carpet or into his shoe. Long before any question of sensation arises, so far as contact with external objects—in this test, either the carpet or the shoe—is concerned, the patient fails to make his muscles obey his will. His foot is thrown out but does not go direct to the mark, it is projected to one side of the object aimed at, or is shot out, as though by explosive force, beyond it ; or sometimes it cannot be extended at all. If any one will take the trouble to study the muscular movements of a spare subject trying to perform these acts, he will, in many cases at least, be able to perceive, by sight and feeling—placing his hand gently on the limb

—that the opposing muscles, extensors and flexors, adductors and abductors, internal and external rotators, and the like, not only fail to act in co-ordination, but are very differently affected by the nerve force projected along the motor nerves of the limb. Only certain muscles will be strongly energized, though the will is acting powerfully, and the endeavour to touch the object be maintained for a time. Some muscles will be spasmodically contracted with a tonic result, having a tendency to run into cramp, while others are affected with an irregular impulse, trembling, twitching, or being even thrown into clonic convulsions. If these phenomena were always present, or still more, if they always appeared in the same muscles, it would be easy to explain the condition on the hypothesis that certain motor branches of the nerves supplying the limb were the seats of mechanical block, and that the nerve force projected from the lower centre at the bidding of the higher automatic and still higher cerebral centres, finding resistance offered on certain lines of nerves, passed off on other lines. The condition is not, however, by any means constant. At times an ataxic patient will walk well, at others he can scarcely stand. One day he can perform almost any desired movement, while on another he can scarcely do anything in an orderly fashion. Nor is it possible to connect the variations which take place in his power of co-ordination with the mental or body state. At least, I have failed to establish any such connection. Sometimes I have thought a patient more orderly in his movements when he was a little depressed; at others, when he was brightest. Treating many cases at the same time, I have observed a tendency on the part of each and all of them—although not in communication, even in my waiting-rooms—to be at their worst on the same day, and have naturally looked to the weather, or the state of the atmosphere, as regards temperature, moisture, and electrical conditions for an explanation. I cannot say that I have succeeded in discovering any connection. The only observation I have been able to make is that there is evidently a tendency to periodicity in the variations, not by direct recurrence of the phenomenon at rhythmical periods, but rather in short series of minor variations. Just as the tide rises or falls by ascending or descending series of waves, some ninth or tenth, or it may be fifth, being the larger, so does an ataxic patient get better or worse in the progress of his disease; and it is not very difficult, by keeping a careful record of any considerable number of these cases seen, at very short intervals—daily, if practicable—to determine whether the tide, in even indolent cases, is rising or falling, so far as the malady as a whole is concerned. Sometimes patients, who suppose themselves to be mending, and who are thought to be "doing well," are really losing ground, and not slowly; while every now and again it happens that a patient who suffers very severely at certain periods, and is greatly alarmed, while his medical attendant is probably hopeless, is, in fact, making a tide-like progress towards health, with terribly long waves, which fall back to return, not in a steady advance proportioned to their recoil, but in a broken series of small advances.

The point I am anxious to bring out is this. If

the real cause of ataxia were the sclerosis found after death, the clinical history would be altogether different. There would be a distinct stage of irritation during the early days of the deposit, before it became sufficient in quantity to create a block; then there would be a gradual and steady paralysis. The only variations possible would depend on occasional congestions of the cord or its meninges, and such variations of pressure as *can* take place in the cerebro-spinal fluid. If there were mechanical obstruction by deposit in a particular part of the cord, or on the lines of certain nerve-trunks or branches, it would not be here to-day and gone to-morrow! It is certainly not sclerosis of the posterior or the antero-lateral columns of the cord which produces the want of co-ordination. I have had under my observation more than one case of undoubted tabes spinalis —not of my own diagnosis be it understood—in which sensation has been perfectly restored, and yet the motor power is now almost at it lowest ebb, so far as the legs are concerned, in these cases. There has not been a trace of patellar tendon-reflex for years, but the cutaneous reflexes are strongly marked, and when excited cause considerable muscular contractions.

What, then, is the explanation of the etiology of tabes, which I have to submit? Briefly this. I believe the disease to be at the outset a disorderly vibration of the nerve cells or fibres, and in the end an arrest of vibration altogether. The first organic cause is, I think, a nutritive change in the neurilemma; and in the syphilitic type of the disease, I believe, the specific inflammatory action followed by deposit, extends along the course of the nerve sheaths, ascending to the centre from the chancre. The nerves involved in the induration around a chancre are demonstrably shown to be the seat of perverted cell growth. The researches of Cornil support this view. He says : "The nerve fasciculi which pass into the indurated tissue of a chancre, and which are surrounded by a connective tissue infiltrated with small round cells, are inflamed in their laminated sheaths, the connective tissue which accompanies the vessels between the nerve fibres in the interior of the fasciculi being also inflamed. Thus, in the examination of a chancre removed by Mauriac from Case V., I have been able to study transverse and longitudinal sections of nerve fasciculi. The laminated sheath was separated ; the flat cells between the laminæ were larger and more swollen than normal, or were replaced by numerous elongated, oval, and small cells. In another examination of a chancre, which had been treated by osmic acid, immediately after its removal, the nerve fibres were also normal. I should say, however, in these examinations, I have not searched for the ultimate terminations of the nerves in the papillæ. The inflammation, the separation of the sheath of the nerve fasciculi by cells of a new formation in the tissue of the chancre, is not accompanied with pain. This neuritis without pain is a curious circumstance."*

Tabes may be originated by spinal irritation of any kind, either mechanical, as in a fall, or by cold, as in meningitis. However, the thickening of the envelope

* "Syphilis," by V. Cornil, Professor in the Faculty of Medicine of Paris. Translated by Sims and White, Philadelphia. H. Kimpton, 1882.

of the nerve or cord is produced, it has the effect of preventing orderly vibration of the adjacent nerve elements, with the result of disturbing and impairing the function of co-ordination. The motor impulse comes down in all integrity from the higher centres; but one of the hammers, so to say, strikes a wire which is out of adjustment and vibrates irregularly, and the musical chord produced is defective, because its component notes are out of tune! The disturbance set up being always located in, or springing from, one segment of the cord or one series of nerves, is likely to be fairly constant in its effects, but there is no more reason why these should not vary from day to day and hour to hour, than that a piano, which is out of tune, should not produce the strangest vagaries of disorderly sound. In short, I believe the cause of the malady to be a disturbance of that orderly vibration which is essential to nerve action and function, whether in the posterior, lateral, or anterior, columns of the cord, or in the nerves that transmit impressions from the periphery or carry down motor impulses from the centres to the muscles. By-and-by, the consequence of this perversion of function is to impair nutrition, and the cells and fibres atrophy, the surrounding connective tissue proliferates, and the disease becomes incurable. Up to this point, however, it is remediable by excitation to normal exercise, and consequent healthy nutrition, and in the process of the cure by re-education nerve-vibration is an accessory remedy ready to hand. It controls the disorder, changes the state, and helps to re-establish that mobility of the nervous elements which is essential to health. Moreover, it is itself a powerful agent in the work of education by restoring not merely vibration but rhythm.

Nerve-vibration is of value also as a means of giving precision to diagnosis by enabling the physician to discover the locality of the disturbance. For example, he passes the percuteur, with the pointed hammer, or the hard brush, gently over the surface of the limb, commencing at the toes and working upwards ; when the nerves are healthy there is no disturbance, but the moment the point of the percuteur touches the skin over a morbid nerve a reflex action commences, and in a few seconds, or longer—as the nerve centres may be more or less out of tune—the muscles which can be reflexly contracted from that particular spot are thrown into a state of spasm. It will be easy to see how, with a fair knowledge of the nervous system, the clinical investigator may trace the disturbed branches to their trunks, and finally up to the cord. The process is at once intensely interesting in itself, and of highly practical value to the patient, because when the particular tracts which are affected have been clearly made out, the vibration may be so applied as to act on these and these alone.

This brings me by a somewhat discursive route back to the practical question, how "to allay morbid irritability?" Granted that I am right in my hypothesis of the sort of disturbance which occurs in tabes spinalis and the allied maladies, ranging from cataleptic hysteria to tetanus, it follows that in so far as the irritability—whether it manifest itself in jerkings, or clonic or tonic spasms—is the result of disorderly vibration, this may be reduced by overpowering the disorder with order. The manner of operating is to apply the flat-headed hammer, if we have to deal with a deeply-placed or large nerve sheath, the pointed hammer if the nerve be superficial or small, the hard brush if several nervous filaments lying close together are affected, or the disk if the area of superficial disturbance be very large ; and to keep up the percussion until the jerking, twitching, or spasm, reflexly excited by the vibration subsides. Either of two courses may be pursued :—1. The percussion, which should always be as light as will suffice to produce the phenomenon, may cease the moment the muscles are contracted, being recommenced when they relax ; or (2) it may be maintained during the spasm. There is a considerable drain of nerve force from the centres when the latter course is pursued. The conditions of expediency will vary with the cases under treatment; but I am inclined to think it is generally well to stop the percussion when the muscles are fully contracted. They will then relax, and after an interval we may repeat the vibration ; sometimes this repetition will need to take place three or four times.

If the patient be in fairly good general health, the treatment may be expedited by continuing the percussion during the spasm, and directing him to resist the effects of vibration. This is perfectly easy to do. The spasm is purely reflex, and the moment a motor impulse is sent through the automatic centre by or from the cerebral centre, the spasm ceases. The educationary process consists in this exercise, the effort being to subdue the insubordinate lower centre, and discipline it to obey the higher centres. It is like drilling a stupid, or stubborn recruit. Nor is the drill merely functional. By the law of development through the environment—the great law of Nature—function precedes organization, and it is not only possible to improve the nutrition of a nerve centre by exercising it, but actually to restore its cells and fibres to health, just as you may promote the growth of brain cells by education.* In this way it is that irritability may be allayed by nerve-vibration, the cause of irritability—that is, disorderly vibration—being rectified by the controlling, subduing, and disciplinary effect of the mechanical vibration applied from without. If I am right, the disorderly state we have to treat must be the same, whether the cause of the disturbance is the irritation set up by a patch of deposit creeping along the sheath of a nerve and gradually encroaching on the space necessary for the oscillatory movements of the essential nerve elements in vibration, or a disturbed and irregular activity of the cells or fibres from any other cause—*e.g.*, the excessive mobility of the nerve elements in the female organism, which renders hysteria, and in some states cataleptic hysteria, a physiologically probable form of nerve derangement. It is needless to adduce evidence which will at once occur to the mind of every practitioner in proof of the essential identity of the nerve-state—without reference to its cause—in the several maladies which are characterized by excessive irritability. It follows that the principle of the treatment by vibration

* See a paper on "The Re-education of the Adult Brain," reproduced at p. 94.

must be the same, however greatly the precise mode of its application may need to vary in cases of different class and type.

The following paper relates to an important adjunct to nerve-vibration. The principle of the procedure is applicable to the treatment of other disabilities besides that for which I have here specially recommended its adoption. The method suggested aims at the regeneration of the nerve element by exercise on the basis of the law of development through function. I reproduce it from the *Practitioner* of November, 1881.

"A Note on One 'Symptom' of Locomotor Ataxia.

"The hypothesis of dissolution as propounded by Herbert Spencer and applied by Hughlings-Jackson to the elucidation of morbid phenomena, receives pointed illustration in the pathognomonic symptom, so-called, of locomotor ataxia. The patient cannot preserve his equilibrium, but begins to reel, when his eyes are closed, being unable to stand or walk without the assistance of the sense of sight. Why is this? I reply, because the automatic function of balancing the body and maintaining the erect posture, has been learnt—as all functions which are performed by the co-ordination of muscular movements must be learned before they can be relegated to the domain of the sub-consciousness, and become automatic—by *sight;* and the ataxic subject is reduced by 'dissolution' to the position of a child just learning to stand and walk. He has lost the nervous bases of the organized movements which are essential to the performance of these muscular acts automatically. The records are either isolated from the current of energy ; or obliterated so far as the active vitality of the cells or molecules composing them is concerned, although the germinal points of the latter are not, perhaps, destroyed, and recovery is possible ; or those elements of the brain or cord on which the lessons have been impressed are atrophied, and the records are finally effaced.

"The infant fixes its gaze steadily on some object when it first tries to stand, and it is by the aid of sight it at length succeeds in steadying itself and in balancing the weight its lower limbs have to carry and its vertebral column has to hold upright. The process by which the child learns first to stand and then to walk, is identical with that by which the tight-rope-walker learns to perform his feats of equipoise. In both cases the gaze is centred on a fixed object, and the muscular sense trained to control the movements of the body, so that the direction of the line of sight may not be disturbed. When the child has once acquired the power of standing, the so-called 'muscular sense' is able to balance the body without the aid of sight, and under normal conditions it is as easy to stand or, so far as muscular action is concerned, to walk with the eyes closed as open. When, however, disease of a paralytic type assails the organism, the most recently acquired faculty is the first to be lost. This rule of denudation from the surface downwards governs, as we know, the demoralization of character in brain disease, and the disorganization of function throughout the system. In the particular manifestation of disease called locomotor ataxia—an arbitrary name for an artificially defined combination of phenomena—the power of balancing the body by the muscular sense is lost, and the subject unconsciously falls back on the method of performing the act of standing which he adopted when first learning the process. It is only accidentally, or when the physician applies the test, that the patient becomes aware of his condition. In the case of a blind man who is ataxic, the muscular sense has been so highly developed to compensate for the loss of sight, that it is not easily impaired even by paralytic disease, and therefore, in the case of the blind, the distinctive symptom of ataxia is often wanting, or seems to be so, until an advanced stage of the disease.

"So far as I am aware, this explanation of the characteristic symptom of locomotor ataxia—which I submit is the true one—has not been given in any treatise on the disease. It is important that it should be recognized, because it affords corroborative evidence of the hypothesis of dissolution undoing the work of evolution—that form of evolution which takes place in the individual under educationary influences; and because it supplies a clue to the method of treatment most likely to be effectual in *delaying* the progress, if not even arresting the advance, of organic disease. No one who believes, as I most firmly do, that *all* development is evolutionary, in the Darwinian sense, and that what we designate mind is the function of nervous matter, in part located in the brain and in part in the spinal cord, can refuse to admit that the brain—and if the brain, why not all the other nervous centres ?—may be organically developed or improved by training, through and by the influence of function, just as muscular tissue may be developed and its nutrition promoted by passive or induced movement. In short, the nerve-centres which are the seat of disease in locomotor ataxia, may, at least in the early stages of disease, be stimulated to normal activity and incited to restorative energy by influences exerted through function, if only we take the pains to study the *modus operandi* of function, and to discover how it was originally evolved.

"The functional act of standing was developed first by the aid of sight, and then by the aid of the muscular sense. In locomotor ataxia the muscular sense is abolished, and the subject left to stand and walk again by sight, or, in other words, reduced to the position of a child. Now, heterodox and unphysiological as it may at the first mention be thought, I propose to arrest the decay, or to renew the activity, of the muscular sense, by re-educating the nerve-cells which are sources of this particular form of energy. Of course, when I use the term "muscular sense," I do not for a moment suppose there is any sensation evolved in muscular tissue. All I mean is, that the nerves of sensation are tributary to the co-ordination of muscular acts in a way which seems to make the very muscles themselves appear sensitive. It is a mere figure of speech which may be taken to represent the instant, consensual, almost reflex government of the muscular system, or trained series of muscles, in the automatic performance of combined movements which, have been learned and organized. What I suggest, therefore, is really the stimulation of these nerve-cells —whence springs the so-called "muscular sense" used in standing and walking—by specifically directed excitants. Every patient suffering from a malady which in the most distant or indirect manner points to brain or nerve disease should be tested, not only for the power of standing firmly, but for ability to walk with a slow and firm tread with the eyes closed. If there be the slightest defect in this performance a distinct exercise designed to train this faculty should be directed and perseveringly carried out, with intent to increase the activity and promote the nutrition of the centres which are failing.

"The symptom to which I have alluded is only one of a series indicating a particular malady, but it is one that points directly to the organic lesion from which the disease as a whole proceeds, or in which it mainly consists. By treating the deep cause, through the functional irritation, the disease may, I am convinced by experiment, be delayed, or, as it seems, wholly arrested. As it is, the disorganization proceeds until the sufferer is reduced to the condition of a child, and the power of standing automatically is lost before the existence of the malady is recognized. Dr. Buzzard has done great and lasting service to the interests of early diagnosis in diseases of the cord by popularizing Westphal's test for 'Tendon-Reflex.' There may be little new in my suggestion, that *every* patient should be tried for the power of balancing the body and maintaining the upright position steadily without the aid of sight; but there is at least novelty, if nothing else, in the recommendation of a serious attempt to stimulate the nervous centres to improved nutrition by formal exercises. I make this recommendation as the result of experiment, and with good grounds, for confidence in the effect at which it aims. In any case no harm can be done by trying the treatment I suggest, and I am persuaded that if it be honestly and perseveringly pursued in the early stages of the disease, it will be found beneficial.

"The plan is simply this: the patient is to be directed to stand with his eyes closed in his bath, after pouring a small can of cold water down the spine (in some cases which appeared to be sthenic I have directed the application of a mustard-poultice over the full length of the spine, for ten minutes or a quarter of an hour, until redness was produced, every night, besides the cold douche in the morning), and to persevere in the attempt to do this *steadily* for, at first, a quarter of an hour, and, as his state improves, for half an hour, every morning. He is to be furnished with a chair or rail at hand to which he can cling in case of need, but instructed to avoid using it except in actual danger of falling. When he commences the daily exercise he will probably for some two or three weeks make little progress, but after this time he will begin to be able to stand, and in less than three months, if my results are trustworthy—not only will the symptom, which was regarded as conclusively indicating the existence of an incurable disease, be eliminated from the case, but other symptoms will disappear with it, and the general state of the patient be sensibly improved. I will not say more as to the effect of this treatment; but I will venture to add that it ought to be tried.

"Before leaving the subject of locomotor ataxia, although this brief note has for its topic one symptom only, I should like to embrace the opportunity of saying that marked benefit seems likely to attend the use of mechanical vibrations propagated through the bony column to the spine in the manner desribed by me in a letter to *The Lancet*, October 15, 1881."

Since I wrote this last paragraph, greatly extended experience has confirmed my good opinion of the effects of nerve-vibration in these cases; but I do not now, as has been explained, attack the centres indirectly through the spinal column, so much as directly—in the physiological sense—through their afferent nerves.

On September 23 last, the following brief note appeared in the *British Medical Journal*, on the Locomotor Ataxy of Tabes Dorsalis, or as Sir William Gull has more correctly named it, Tabes Spinalis. Every one must admit the justice of the remark made by Sir William when presiding at the discussion which took place on the subject of this symptom or malady in the International Medical Congress of 1881: "Tabes *Dorsalis* certainly it is not."

"A NOTE ON THE TREATMENT OF LOCOMOTOR ATAXY BY PRECISE NERVE-VIBRATION.

"I do not think the evidence collected, up to this point is sufficient to justify the assertion, that locomotor ataxy can be certainly cured by nerve-vibration; but the large measure of success I have recently obtained in dealing with some very advanced cases of this truly terrible disease, seems to render it incumbent upon me to place the facts before the profession. The cases I have had have all been clearly marked, with entire absence of patellar tendon-reflex, and with the characteristic impairment, in some instances amounting to almost complete loss, of the power of co-ordination. It is not my intention to report these cases at present, as I am anxious to extend the area of observation, both as regards the number of cases and their duration, before committing myself to a final judgment. Meanwhile there are certain clinical facts which may be helpful to others, and ought, therefore, to be communicated. I will try to state them as tersely as possible.

"1. In every instance I find exaggerated reflex irritability on application of the percuteur to the periphery. For example, when it is applied over the anterior tibial (a mixed) nerve, the foot is drawn forcibly up, which never happens in the case of a healthy subject. In some instances the irritability is so great that the legs and feet may be turned or drawn in any direction at pleasure, by vibrating the appropriate afferent branches of the nerves supplying them. No effect is produced by percussing the muscles; the effect follows only precise vibration of the nerves.

"2. This reflex irritability, or excitability, seems to me the real hindrance to the walking; the loss of sensation, which is incident to the malady, being of comparatively secondary importance as regards the disability for locomotion. It is almost invariably confined to the nerves supplying the extensors. I have not in any instance met with more than a slight tendency to cramp in the flexors, and that rarely.

"3. By persisting in the vibration of the irritable nerves, their excitability becomes exhausted; and, in proportion as this happens, they obey the mandate of the will, and voluntary movements, in short, locomotive acts, are possible. Not unfrequently some debility of the nerve-power and depression of energy in the centres follow immediately upon the exhaustion of their irritability; so that for a few hours, or it may be days, the patient complains of stiffness, and, although he may have lost the jerky feeling in his limbs, he cannot move them more readily. They are heavy and powerless. This, however, quickly passes away, and the case is found to have made decided progress. The walking is easier and steadier, and control, generally, more direct and precise. At this stage, not earlier, it may be advantageous to percuss over the spines of the vertebræ, with the view of vibrating the nerve-centres. I do not think it is easy, or in many cases possible, to excite the centres except through their afferent nerves; but after the reflex irritability has been reduced, it then often happens that vibrations, which could not at first be propagated along the motor nerves, can be sent from the centres by percussion immediately, or as nearly as possible, over the latter. I believe it will be found that the mechanical vibrations excited in a nerve by percussion, invariably pass in the direction of its normal activity—in the sensory branch, towards the centre; in the motor towards the periphery. There often seems to be a block, as it were, in the course of a nerve, whether motor or sensory, and, while this lasts, the impulse or impression is diverted, sometimes producing very curious results under vibration by percussion. When the block is broken down by mechanical vibration, the wave again passes in the normal direction. Practically, I do not find much amiss with the sensory nerves. The motor chiefly are at fault.

"4. I have collected almost, though perhaps not quite, enough evidence to show that the syphilitic form of locomotor ataxy, or that which undoubtedly follows syphilitic disease, is not a localized, but a local affection. It is a specific inflammatory extension from the penis along the sheaths of the nerves to the proximate centre, and thence by particular fibres to other parts of the cord. The loss of sexual power which occurs, and which is rapidly followed by the indications of deficient nutritive action in the organs of generation, is the immediate consequence of an interruption, more or less considerable, in the nervous connections, consequent on the affection of the nerve-sheaths. The impairment of control over the bladder and sphincters, causing either diarrhœa or constipation, is contingent on the local progress of the disease, which may generally be traced by the anatomical and physiological communications. It is very instructive to work out the details of a case of this class clinically; and no two cases, in my experience, have been alike, although as a rule they have surface-features of typical resemblance. For example, there is nearly always something wrong with one of the ulnar nerves, not, I believe, as an accident of disseminated sclerosis, but as a specific extension along particular fibres. I am convinced that these cases of syphilitic ataxy ought to be studied apart, and treated as distinct, from the mass of ataxic disease. The two maladies have little, if anything, in common beyond the name; and that is, as regards both, I think, a misnomer. Moreover, the sensory fault is by no means the primary one, as generally supposed.

"5. The sclerosis which occurs in the cord in the syphilitic disease, I believe to be simply inflammatory thickening of a specific character. I do not think we need talk of 'gummata' or 'disseminated sclerosis.' The malady consists in a direct extension of the local disease along the sheaths of particular nervous tracts. Syphilis is, of course, one of the blood-diseases; but I doubt whether syphilitic 'ataxy' falls into that category. The interval which occurs between the healing of a chancre and the appearance of ataxic symptoms may be great; but, if we inquire carefully into the history of cases, we find that there have throughout been indications—very slight it may be—of local nerve disturbance. Nerve-vibration, unquestionably, does much for these cases; and among other effects which it produces, and for which it is well to provide, is that, in the course of the treatment, it every now and again revivifies the syphilitic virus, and thus at once renders it possible, and necessary, to treat the malady *de novo*, even in cases of very long standing, where there has been no thought of active syphilitic poison for years. Whether the mechanical vibration of the nerves, with their thickened sheaths, throws off particles of poisonous exudation which find their way into the current of the blood, as in the breaking down of an old cicatrix which has entangled the virus of rabies, I can only conjecture.

"It seems possible that the nerve-fibres, which have been mechanically blocked by the exudative processes of the specific disease may be, as it were, shaken loose from their entanglement, and thus become again vibratile. Perhaps it is in the course of this breaking up of the 'block' *débris* are thrown into the circulation. However the revival of the original specific disease may be explained, it undoubtedly every now and again occurs.

" I have thus just jotted down briefly, and in no formal sequence, the leading facts which I desire to place on record, and to which I think the attention of the profession ought to be directed. One word only, in conclusion: nerve vibration by percussion is undoubtedly a most useful adjunct to the ordinary treatment of many maladies, and of especial value in the diagnostic study of disease. It will be monstrous if this method be degraded to the level of a 'cure,' by placing percuteurs in the hands of patients, and allowing them to use them for themselves. Great harm will be done in some cases, in others there will be disappointment, and nerve-vibration will be discredited. It is an agency for professional use exclusively; and against its employment by laymen, whether alone or under medical advice, I must most earnestly protest."

TO RELIEVE CEREBRAL AND CEREBRO-SPINAL IRRITATION AND DISTRESS.

I use these terms, *irritation* or *distress*, to indicate the commonest forms of brain and mind trouble, because no others seem to me to express with equal precision the states for which I believe vibration to be a good remedy. Irritation conveys the idea of excitement arising from debility, and distress indicates that labouring and yet consciously ineffective state of the brain-power which constitutes one of the most painful forms of mental misery.

The general remarks offered under the last heading apply, *mutatis mutandis*, to the subject now before us. The treatment for irritability, whether cerebral, cerebro-spinal—in the sense of seeming to pervade the whole nervous axis—or spinal, such as that I have previously discussed, must be essentially the same. It consists of two parts, (1) healthy stimulation and re-education through function ; and (2) rhythmical vibration to subdue tumultuous and irregular vibration of the nervous elements and thus restore order. I should like in this place to cite a case which formed the subject of a short paper which appeared in *Brain*, Part VII. October, 1879, on "Re-education of the Adult Brain." It was suggested by a very interesting and important case narrated by Professor Sharpey in the April number of the same periodical, which recalled to memory one that fell under my own observation many years before.

"In 1858 I was requested to see a daily governess

and teacher of music, who had been suddenly attacked with what was thought to be acute mania. I found a spare, somewhat angular, eccentric looking young woman, aged about 26, in a state of great excitement, hysterical and choreic. Within a few hours—after a paroxysm of considerable violence, during which she talked and sang wildly, and was with difficulty restrained by those around her—she fell into a state verging on suspended animation, which lasted a week. The skin was cold, and presented a dark mottled appearance; the pulse was scarcely perceptible at the wrist; the breathing slow and seldom deep; there seemed to be complete loss of consciousness, and scarcely any trace of sensibility. The muscles were cataleptic, and the extremities dropped slowly when raised. It was barely possible to feed the patient by the mouth, by holding forward the larynx and placing the fluid far back in the pharynx with a spoon, when it seemed to flow down the œsophagus as through a flaccid tube. This condition, which was treated with the interrupted current from the occiput and nape to the hypogastrium, and mustard-poultices down the spine, subsided very gradually. Then came the state I am chiefly interested to describe. There had been an exciting cause for the attack in religious excitement, acting on a nervous system exhausted by protracted toil as a teacher.

"When consciousness began to return, the latest sane ideas formed previous to the illness, mingled curiously with the new impressions received, as in the case of a person awakening slowly from a dream. When propped up with pillows in bed near the window, so that passers in the street could be seen, the patient described the moving objects as 'trees walking;' and when asked where she saw these things, she invariably replied 'in the other gospel.' In short, her mental state was one in which the real and the ideal were not separable. Her recollections on recovery, and for some time afterwards, were indistinct, and, in regard to a large class of common topics which must have formed the staple material of her cerebration up to the period of the attack, memory was blank. Special subjects of thought immediately anterior to the malady seemed to have saturated the mind so completely that the early impressions received after recovery commenced were imbued with them, while the cerebral record of penultimate brain work, in the life before the morbid state, was, as it were, obliterated. For example: although this young woman had supported herself by daily duty as a governess, she had no recollection of so simple a matter as the use of a writing implement. When a pen or pencil was placed in her hand, as it might be thrust between the fingers of a child, the act of grasping it was not excited, even reflexly: the touch or sight of the instrument awoke no association of ideas. The most perfect destruction of brain tissue could not have more completely effaced the constructive effect of education and habit on the cerebral elements. This state lasted some weeks, and the "recollection" of what had been "forgotten," to use conventional terms, was slow and painful, needing, or, as I would now say, *seeming* to require, a process of re-education as distinct as (though, I judge, less prolonged than) that which proved necessary in the case detailed by Professor Sharpey. In the end recovery was mentally and physically satisfactory.

"I cannot assume that anything in these two narratives (Professor Sharpey's and my own) will strike the practical psychologist as novel, or of even unfrequent occurrence. The clinical aspect of such cases has been sketched times without number. Nevertheless, they present features of interest, as viewed from an etiological stand-point, which may be worthy of more than a passing notice.

"Either of three conditions may, I believe, be set up by brain disturbance, or disease, causing 'loss of memory':—1. Complete destruction of cerebral cells; 2. Withering or blighting, which amounts to obliteration of the cells without destruction of their nuclei (I use the term *nucleus*, here and throughout, in a non-physiological sense, simply to designate the seat of life in a cell, whatever that may be); 3. A suspension of function without arrest of nutrition, as though a particular area of the cerebral organism were simply thrown out of the circuit of energy.

"In the first event there will be final effacement of the records of ideation. So far as the cells destroyed are concerned, they and their properties are lost for ever. If the functions previously performed by these strata or tracts reappear, it must be because some other part of the brain has taken up the business vicariously—as I believe is possible with nearly every function or manifestation of mental energy. In the second event, when the cells are withered, but the nuclei remain, a new crop of cells may spring from the parent organism, and after a lapse of time sufficient for development, the educationary record will reappear, the seed reproducing its kind, plus the impress of training and ideation. It may be that there will need to be so much re-education as to cultivate the new growth, and perhaps a re-impression of purely objective ideas, but it may, and probably in the majority of instances does, happen that the new cells will be developed with all the characteristics of the old. In the third event, recovery may occur instantly, almost at any moment, if the obstacle to communication be overcome or break down in convalescence, so that the isolated, but scarcely injured, congeries of brain cells may again be energized. I speak of brain cells instead of 'nerve-molecules,' because, accepting the vibration theory, it must be assumed that the vibrating particles are cellular vital organisms.

"Supposing the states I have described to exist, I venture to suggest that the development of a new crop of cells from denuded germs or nuclei will account for the facility with which re-education, in cases like that described by Professor Sharpey, reproduces *knowledge*, even at a period of life when it is not easy to learn, What the new training and teaching does is not so much to impart information as to foster the growth of a new crop from the old seed, just as an after-crop may be procured by breaking up an over-stocked soil and applying the stimulus of manure. It is always possible that in the first process of instruction more seed may have been sown than germinated. Some good mental seed doubtless falls on barren ground, and it is perhaps due to the vitality and subsequent germination of this

G

seed, ideas we do not seem to have cultivated deepen as the years go on.

"Meanwhile I fancy it is as the progeny of old nuclei the physical bases of a revived memory are restored during general recovery in cases of the class before us. It seldom happens that the re-educating process needs to be very explicit or prolonged. Far less teaching than was required to implant the knowledge in the first instance will cause it to reappear. In cases where the cells only are destroyed and their centres of vitality remain, it may even happen that the mere re-establishment of health will suffice to bring about complete mental restoration. When the new cells grow, the old memories will be revived. This is what takes place in ordinary cases, when, although no especial pains are taken to re-educate, 'lost' knowledge returns. The completeness of the recovery will probably depend on the vigour of the first growth, and is doubtless governed by the same law which determines permanence or tendency to revert to an old type in the propagation of recently impressed or acquired qualities of species or family. Ideas, or an organic tendency to form particular conceptions, are certainly transmitted from parent to child. The cells first developed in a fœtal cerebrum are probably imbued with the qualities and properties of the brains of the mother and father, in different proportions. The transmission of germs of mental character which slumber through one generation and awaken with all their ancestral energy in the next [Atavism of mind] is a recognized fact. It will therefore probably happen that the new crop does not at first present all the features of that which was blighted by disease, but develops part of its characteristics later on. Thus vigorous health at an advanced period of life will sometimes produce a perfecting of the recovery commenced, but not consummated, years before.

"Cases of the first and third class are very likely to be confounded in practice. Final destruction may be assumed when, perhaps, a tract has been isolated without being destroyed. In this way I venture to think hopeless 'dementia' is occasionally diagnosed, when what has happened is the disconnection, or throwing out of the circuit of cerebral energy, of a particular tract or stratum of elements: and, unless wātched, partial recovery, susceptible of treatment, may happen without being observed and helped at the critical moment.

"Treatment for the first class of cases is valueless; for the second, the cure must consist in the reproduction of brain cells, or rather, as I have suggested, the development of a new crop from the denuded nuclei of blighted cells. The so-called 're-education' is only in a limited, and scarcely physiological sense, educationary. It is a repetition of the training, not so much to teach as to stimulate the growth of new organic elements from pre-existent germs imbued with formative forces and characteristics which must themselves determine the physico-mental result. If new cells *are* produced, they will be found already educated—that is, endowed with inherited characteristics which constitute the physical bases of memory. The educated germ naturally produces an educated cell. Upon this hypothesis rests the whole theory of heredity, species, and transmission.

"In the third class of cases, recovery occurs as an

accident of treatment, except when in the presence of a constitutional cachexia like syphilis, specific medication may remove the grip of disease which, so to say, holds the mental organism in fetters that its energy cannot break. It will, I think, be often found that the seemingly permanent losses of memory which occur after acute disease are due to the isolation of special strata of cerebral tissue by the stasis of syphilitic or gouty disease. Mercury, iodide of potassium, or colchicum, may in this way serve as 'memory-powder,' and work a cure.

"The two points I am chiefly anxious to place on record, without any claim to novelty of suggestion are—first, that what is called re-education is often simply the fostering of a natural growth—never harmful unless overdone, but of less value than may at first sight be supposed; second, that, in the absence of special andications that what seems to be helpless dementia is actually what it seems—*i.e.*, a physical destruction of brain-cells—it is always *possible* the patient may recover, and therefore never justifiable to write a case off as incurable, and leave it to drift unnoticed and unhelped."

M. Ribot, in his interesting work on "Disorders of Memory," has laid some stress on the explanation I offered, in this little paper, of the physical, or, if anyone please, let him say, the *pathological* cause of morbid irritability, distress, and loss of memory. This case occurred nearly five-and-twenty years ago, before the method of treatment for which I am endeavouring to obtain the consideration of the profession had suggested itself, and even as late as 1879 I had not had such experience with nerve-vibration in cases of mind-troubles as would justify the recommendation of its use. I have now the solid ground of fact to go upon, and without affirming its sufficiency in all cases, to allay the morbid irritability which constitutes mania, to supply the strength of purpose and clearness of thought that lie at the base of true intellectual vigour, or to rouse the consciousness out of that lethargy which in too many cases of brain-disorder merges in the apathy of dementia, paralysis, and death, I may venture to say that there are few instances in which the patient will not be benefited and the power of other remedies and modes of treatment augmented, by vibration precisely and judiciously applied.

The way vibration causes, or helps, recovery in this class of cases is, doubtless, by exciting the cerebral centres to orderly exercise, and by energizing, and, as it were, methodizing the activity of, the centres and nervous apparatus of the organs of special sense. Precisely what can be done for the cord may be done for the brain. The organs of the senses severally represent the distal extremities of afferent nerves, and to these particularly the vibration should be applied. It is not very difficult, though in some cases it calls for special skill and adaptation on the part of the operator to administer the remedy. For example, in appealing to the optic centre through the eye, it is necessary to apply the percuteur in such way that the retina may be thrown into vibrations of greater force and amplitude than those which agitate it in the performance of its specific functions. Doubtless all light is vibratile, and the reflection of light from the surfaces of external objects, in the presence of the organ of vision in such way that they are *seen,* acts on the rods and cones of the retinal expansion of the optic nerve *mechanically.*

A sharp blow on the eyeball produces a sensation of seeing light! The vibrations propagated to the retina by a scene or picture of any kind are carried back to the proper centre through and by the optic nerve. Certain changes, of which we know no more definitely than we know of the changes which take place in the centres of the cord in the process of reflex-action, are effected in the visual centre, and the centres which are, so to say, the organs of the consciousness, become cognisant of the impression formed or received. To stimulate this—the visual or optic—centre, and relieve its irritability, to give it tone, or to rouse it when inert—not for its own sake only or chiefly, but for the sake of the mental faculty of sight that stand behinds it, and of which it is the representative and organ of relation—and above all—perhaps in and by—these processes, to improve its nutrition, I apply the disc with exceeding lightness of hand to the closed eyelid, and vibrate for a few seconds only at a time with the highest practicable speed. To secure this effect the battery with the percuteur must be in full working power, and the screw which stands nearest to the hinge or pivot of the vibrator (A, Fig. 2, page 58) must be adjusted to come into play while the distant one is withdrawn from electro-magnetic contact. The operation is one of extreme delicacy, but it is sufficiently easy with ordinary care, and the effects gained should be agreeable to the patient as well as beneficial to his case. Optic neuritis does not contra-indicate the treatment, but is in fact relieved by it. The arterioles are made to contract, and the turgid capillaries relieved of the blood-pressure, while their tone is restored.

In cases of commencing atrophy nutrition may be improved by gentle vibration, administered, as I have said, for a few seconds only at a time with short intervals of rest, the whole operation not being prolonged beyond five minutes. This may be done daily with the best results, both as regards the optic affection and the brain as a whole in the relation of cerebral function to sight—mental sight, dreams of sight, thoughts of sight, and every part or phrase of the intellectuality in which body or mind-vision are involved or concerned. So, again, with the auditory centres, the disc applied over the meatus will act first on the membrane of the tympanum mechanically and through the medium of the apparatus of hearing in its entirety on the faculty and sense of audition, both physical and mental.

It is not necessary to go further into details. After a very few personal experiments with the percuteur, the operator will see how with disc, hammer, brush, or bent arm rod, he can communicate mechanical vibrations to the nose, tongue, palate, and thus act on any afferent nerve he pleases, and through the natural line of communication upon the centre behind. The point to be remembered is, that the influence exerted is twofold ; first on the organ of sense, and then on the cerebral centre which takes cognizance of the effect, and performs the mental act of perception within. It is not necessary to remind the physiological physician, that whatever there may be behind matter, it is only with the morbid organism the medical practitioner has to deal, and for him mind is brain-function ; and thoughts, and feelings, and ideas, and emotions, and beliefs are simply forms of *physical* activity into which particular parts of the brain are thrown, to which they are or may be excited, and which it is necessary to excite for exercise and nutrition, and to bring under control or order. I must leave the profession to judge for itself how far vibration is likely to prove useful in special affections of the eye, the ear, and other organs of special sense. For myself I believe that certain diseases of sight and *some* forms of deafness may be benefited by its influence; but although I have seen good results in cases of this class, I am not specialist enough to carry the application of nerve-vibration into many provinces of possible usefulness with the precision required.

Before leaving this great subject of brain and special sensory nerve-vibration, I will take the opportunity offered to bring under the notice of practitioners two instruments which I find of great clinical value in testing the daily state. The first is a differential spirit thermometer, constructed* so as to admit of the application of an air-ball to opposite parts of the head. The scale is so arranged that 100 divisions represent one degree Fahr. The diagram (Fig. 7) will make the use of the instrument apparent at a glance. The second I have called a strabismometer, because it measures in fiftieths of an inch the rectification necessary to make a pointer appear to lie accurately upon a double line, first when looked at steadily with two eyes, and afterwards with one eye and then with the other, the head being kept in the same position during the few moments occupied by the experiment. This also is a very simple instrument, as will be seen by Fig. 8.

* Negretti & Zambra.

It affords a ready means of measuring convergence and divergence, which I find to be a good indication of the strength or weakness of the muscles

FIG. 7.

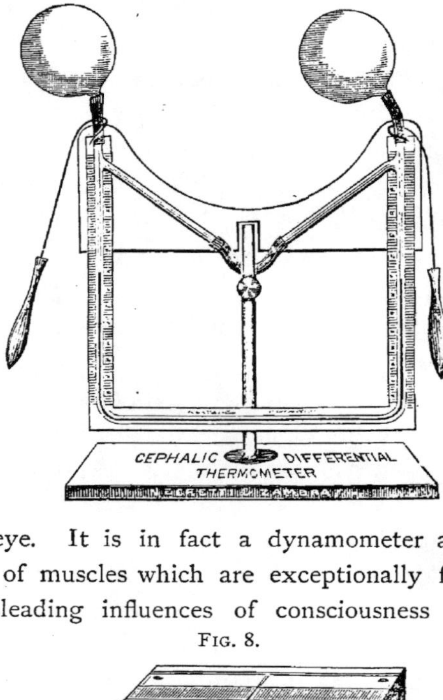

of the eye. It is in fact a dynamometer applicable to a set of muscles which are exceptionally free from the misleading influences of consciousness and the

FIG. 8.

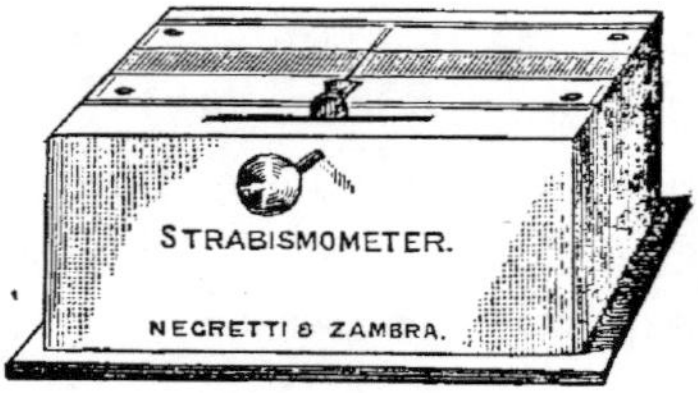

will. I am loth to leave a part of the subject, and a class of maladies, in which I am particularly interested, but I do not feel that the facts I have as yet been able to collect are sufficient to justify more than an appeal to the profession to test nerve-vibration for the remedying of mental and special-sensory disorders and disturbances with especial hopefulness, caution, and care.

To Improve the Vaso-motor State.

I do not think we attach sufficient importance to the vaso-motor state. Setting aside such degeneration of the vascular coats as must cause the vessels to be permanently rigid and contracted, or to be irremediably lax and dilated in consequence of the final destruction of muscular fibres—a very extreme but possible state of matters—every variety of abnormal condition of the arterioles, ranging from spasmodic contraction, almost tetanic, as I believe, despite the notion about tonic spasms occurring only in voluntary muscles, to utter loss of contractability and very nearly complete loss also of elasticity—may be caused by purely functional faults in the innervation of the vessels from irritability or torpor of the vaso-motor system of nerves. Vulpian, of Paris, is probably the only man who has approximately well studied this subject. It is most painfully neglected in English pathology—the pathology of *existing* disease—and is scarcely ever intelligently applied in practice. There is less to marvel at in the last-mentioned than in the other phase, of this omission. Beyond giving a little strychnia or nux vomica, or one or more of some half a dozen so-called "tonics," we have no remedy at command which will go directly to the root of the evil and act specifically on the vaso-motor system. If I am not greatly mistaken, precise nerve-vibration is destined to prove of signal value in this respect. In *The Lancet* of June 10, 1882, I published a few notes of cases intended to illustrate the effect of this treatment on the vaso-motor system. I will here reproduce them with the remark that although I am as sceptical as any one of my readers or critics can possibly be of the value of the sphygmograph as a recording instrument—in fact, I fear it is open to the heavy charge which lies at the door of statistics, namely, that you can show or prove anything with it—I do think in the instances submitted, and in many others I could adduce, the changes indicated by the pulse tracings have been borne out by the improvement in the general state, setting aside the relief afforded in respect to special symptoms.

"A. B., aged forty, consulted me for a highly nervous condition, characterized by a strange mixture of agaraphobia and claustrophobia, with occasional presence of sugar in the urine. I will not anticipate the full report which I may hereafter publish of this case, but simply say that it may be set down as one of long standing and serious neurasthenia. The pulse, taken Dec. 23, 1881, was as below.

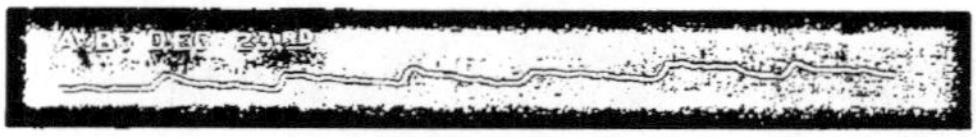

" The case was treated in the usual way with tonics, &c., until Feb. 21, when the general symptoms being in no sensible degree relieved, the patient came to London, and I commenced nerve-vibration. At this date (Feb. 21) I took the following tracing, which

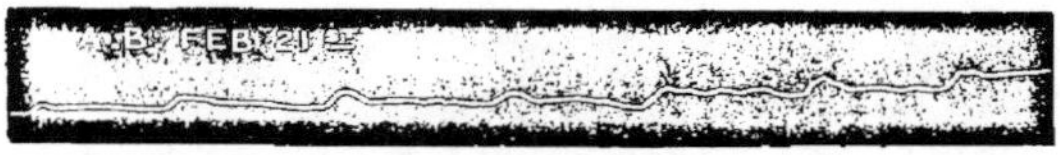

certainly showed no improvement. The percussion was administered daily until March 7, when he left town relieved of all his troublesome symptoms. The last tracing, taken on March 6,

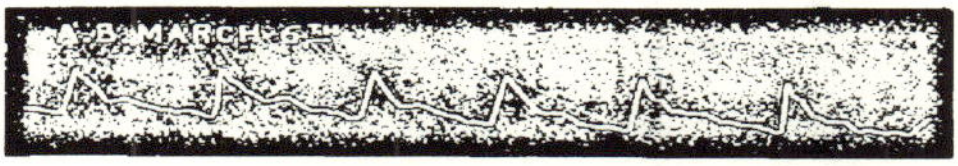

shows a very nearly normal pulse. On April 3, when this patient happened to be in London for a day, he presented himself, improved in general health, and without any return of his old symptoms, a pulse tracing giving the following result :—

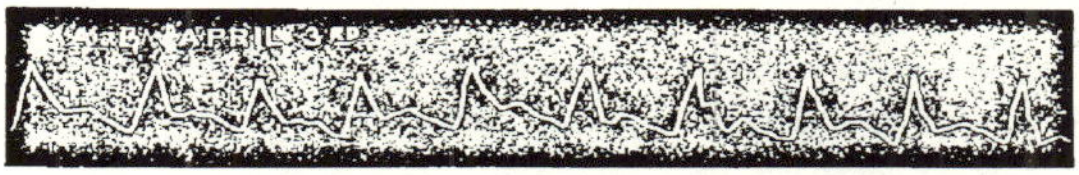

"C. D., aged thirty-seven, with lateral sclerosis, total abolition of patellar tendon-reflex, and so much ataxy as to render walking difficult, a lurching gait, and general unsteadiness, gave the following pulse tracing on April 4 before commencing treatment. On April 12

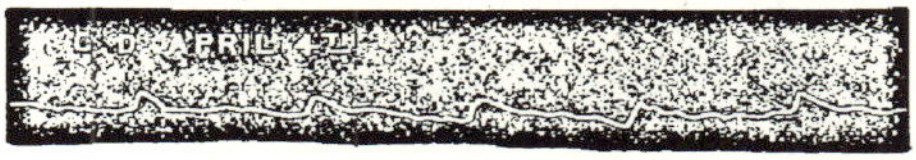

I took the next tracing. The following was taken

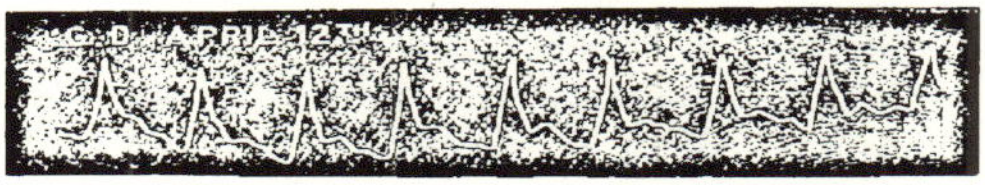

on April 25 :—

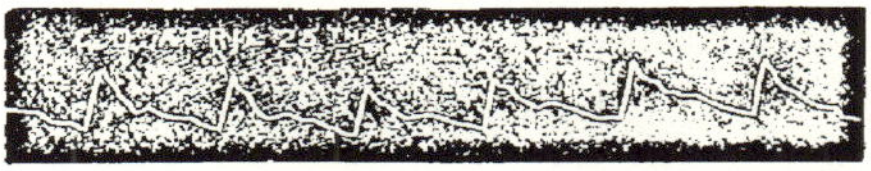

On May 5 the patient left me, walking steadily, automatically, and in a straight line, his health being improved, and the symptoms of his malady generally relieved or in abeyance. The pulse record was then as below :—

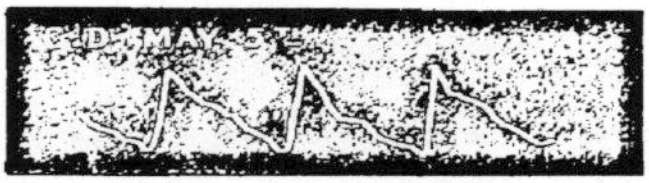

"I will only give one additional instance of this vasomotor improvement. E. F. had suffered from neurasthenia for some seven or eight years, and had been worse for eighteen months. He was intensely nervous, shunned society, and started at the least sound. On March 16, before commencing treatment by nerve-vibration, his pulse tracing was as follows :—

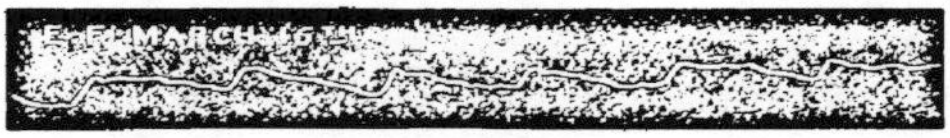

"On March 21 a tracing gave this result :—

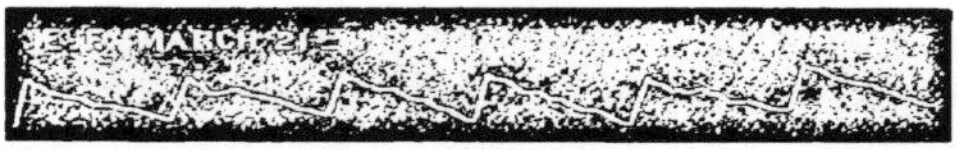

"On April 3 this patient left me practically well, with a pulse tracing which explained the improvement thus :—

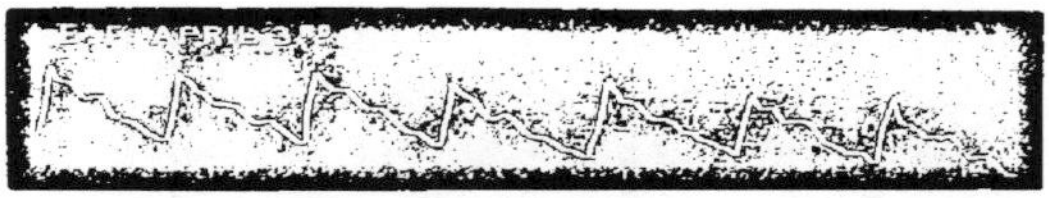

I then wrote, and I would now repeat :—

"I do not wish to lay greater stress on the clinical value of the records taken by the sphygmograph in consulting practice than may be justly due. For myself I would not willingly dispense with the aid afforded by that instrument in judging of the actual state of my patients.

I am careful to apply it under, as nearly as possible, the same conditions of pressure and adjustment on each occasion, and I regard as important *only* the angle formed by the up-stroke and the decline, together with the *relative* proportional amplitude of the waves on the descending line as compared with the height of the up-stroke, whatever that may be. I think, however much we may differ as to the significance of the tracings given above, it will be conceded that the effect of the treatment upon the vaso-motor centre must in each instance have been marked. To this influence I attribute, in a conspicuous degree, the change effected in the general health as well as the amelioration of the particular symptoms."

The researches of MM. Dastre and Morat, to which allusion was made in *The Lancet* of August 19 last, show that vaso-motor activity may be excited from a considerable distance in point of anatomical situation. I have beyond question affected the vessels of the face, and, inferentially, I judge also those of the brain, by percussion over the anterior tibial nerve. It is, however, easy, and therefore justly idle, to multiply mere assertions. The profession will do wisely to make this phase of the subject—namely, the effect of nerve-vibration on the vaso-motor system—one of special observation. I venture to think we are on the eve of important discoveries in relation to this matter, though it will probably be necessary to develop nerve-vibration to a state of very high efficiency before its full benefits can be obtained. I will content myself by enumerating the effects which I have been able to produce in the course of direct endeavours to influence the vaso-motor system by vibrating distant nerves, particularly those of the forearm and of the lower leg and foot. It is curious—it may be an anomaly in my experience—that I have not been able to produce decided results by vibrating over the cervical region, or on the face and head. The results gained and immediately following percussion, in some instances lasting from twelve to twenty-four hours, in others passing off more rapidly, have been marked diminution of conjunctival congestion and increased mobility of the pupils, a healthier and clearer complexion, and better colour of the skin generally, cessation of local perspirations, relief of the feeling of chilliness, of formication, and of tingling, in the skin, the remedy of certain forms of sleeplessness—certain forms only, and I must admit that I do not yet quite understand what these precisely are—increase of mental power and clearness, conversely, relief of mental depression, &c. Most, if not all, of these effects, will be recognized as being direct results of change in the condition of the blood-vessels. Among the more permanent effects produced few have been so marked as the rapid cure of acne, even in cases of long standing; no new spots appearing after a few applications of the percuteur, and the old ones dying rapidly away. Meanwhile the tone and colour of the skin is, as I have said, considerably improved. If I were not restrained by anxiety to avoid overstating my case, I might adduce other tokens of amendment in the general state, which must, I am convinced, also be ascribed to influences exerted on the vaso-motor system, such as the rapid taking up of bile pigment from the skin, in cases which have come under treatment jaundiced by old-standing liver disease. I have not had any opportunity of testing the effect of the remedy in discolorations and affections of the skin generally, but I am exceedingly anxious that it should be thus tested, as I anticipate great results from its use in this important specialty of practice.

The administration, to produce vaso-motor effects, should, I think, be made with the hammer or hard brush, and by preference to distant nerve vessels of some size, rather than locally, though for skin troubles it may be desirable, in addition to this special nerve-vibration, to throw the whole network of subcutaneous nerves into vibration by means of the large disc or the brush, passed slowly over the region of the morbid sensation or appearance. For this purpose the force of the percussion should be very small, the percuteur being held with a light hand. When vibrating large branches of nerves, particularly if somewhat deeply set, it may be necessary to make firm pressure, but the protecting vulcanite tube, through which the hammer passes (D, Fig. 2, p. 58) should be carefully adjusted by screwing, so that the hammer may have full play and strike the skin with its entire force.

NEURASTHENIA.

I have no intention of dwelling upon the pathology of this most distressing malady, though I should like to contend that it is, in the outset at least, a purely functional disorder, consisting in disturbance of the rhythm of the vibration of the nerve elements, such as that which is apt to be set up by slight concussion of the spine in a railway accident. The agitation, consequent upon the first disturbance, whatever it may be, grows worse as time passes, and in the issue organic disease may be induced. I think it is of the highest practical moment to recognize the essential identity of neurasthenia with the group of affections commonly classed together as traumatic—chiefly because they fall first under the observation of the surgeon, . The "railway spine" may be taken as an example of the multitude of differing and yet mutually resembling affections of which I speak. This malady, properly so called, is not the result of accident or of any coarse lesion of the cord, but is set up by the persistent causal injury of frequent railway travelling. The cord is subject to long continuing, or often repeated, vibrations, which are propagated up the line of the axis of the cord. The effect of these vibrations is, I believe, to "polarize" the cord, and to give its fibres a tendency to longitudinal vibration, or, in other words, to form a habit of vibrating in a way that first enfeebles and then disorganizes the nervous structure. The well-known symptoms of neurasthenia spinalis are as nearly as possible those of "railway spine"—with a difference—which difference rather emphasizes the atonic features of the malady. All affections of this class, whether proceeding from shock, persistent vibration in one direction, or other debilitating causes—for example, excessive excitement of the lower segments of the cord in sexual abuse, and particularly masturbation—are, I believe, essentially disorders of a mechanical kind, and the degeneration which takes place in the nervous structure is secondary.

I have had very remarkable cases of rapid recovery under nerve-vibration after confirmed neurasthenia extending over many years. The intense neuralgia which often, though not always, attends spinal neurasthenia, is not unfrequently much relieved or even wholly removed by one or two vibrations, and the intense tenderness which is generally found at one or two points in the range of the spinous processes, is quickly put to flight in one or other of the manners described in the section "In the Relief of Pain."

I will only refer to the first of the three cases of which I have given sphygmographic tracings at page 107; and I mention another in which nerve-vibration, administered daily for a fortnight, removed a neuralgia of this class, involving entire disability for exercise during several years. The periods which have elapsed since the completion of these cases are now sufficiently long to place beyond question the important point of permanency in the cures, for such I may truly call them. I may remark here, as I have elsewhere, that all my cases have been those of men, and that I have done everything in my power to prevent being deceived myself or misleading others.

In the treatment of neurasthenia I generally percuss the spinous processes with the flat hammer, and apply the percuteur also over the interspaces, about an inch on each side of the spinous processes, so as to vibrate the roots of the nerves. I have not yet had any case of neurasthenia, uncomplicated with syphilitic or other severe disease—and I have had many very severe cases of long duration, which have exhausted other forms of treatment, under the best diagnosticians and most able therapeutists both here and on the Continent—that has not yielded to steady vibration for a fortnight. The full effects of the remedy have not in all cases shown themselves until after the treatment has ceased, though there has always been some amendment during the period of daily vibration, but afterwards the gain has been rapid and the recovery evidenced by an unmistakable return to health, without medicine or supplementary treatment of any kind. I cannot speak too strongly of the success of the treatment in cases of the class I am now endeavouring to describe. Nerve-vibration should undoubtedly be tried in all cases of spinal weakness, with or without pain, and whatever the "cause" of the malady be. In extremely neuralgic cases it may be well to begin vibration with the brush, then to use the disc, and after the pain and tenderness have ceased, which will generally happen in a few days, to complete the treatment by percussion with the flat hammer over the spinous processes and the flat or pointed hammer between them. For the relief of spinal neuralgia, I can recommend the remedy with perfect confidence and without reserve. The theory of its action was embodied in a letter to *The Lancet*, which I subjoin. It appeared October 19, 1881:—

"A NEW TREATMENT FOR CERTAIN FORMS OF NEURASTHENIA SPINALIS.

"Some months ago you were good enough to publish a paper in which I introduced to the notice of the profession in England the results obtained, so far as I had then obtained any results, in the course of a long-pending inquiry with respect to nerve-vibration, and the treatment of pain in certain neuralgic states by mechanical vibration. It may be remembered that I announced the conclusions at which I had arrived quite tentatively and under protest, in consequence of a claim to the discovery made by M. Boudet de Paris, in one of the French journals. I am not yet able to say that pain *is* relieved by any mechanical vibration which I have been able to apply, although the frequency of the *post hoc* in a considerable number of cases leads me to think it will hereafter prove to be *propter hoc*.

"Meanwhile, I have lighted on a new, and seemingly successful, mode of treating certain forms of neurasthenia spinalis, and, at the risk of being charged with precipitation, I feel bound to place the facts on record. They are briefly these. Persons who travel much by railway and suffer from what has been termed the 'railway spine,' which is neurasthenic though neurosthenic, and others who are affected with spinal debility, the result of exhaustion from any of a variety of causes—ranging from mechanical shock to sexual excess—and who may be supposed to be the subjects of a loss of tone or elasticity in the fibres of the spinal cord, are not only relieved of their strangely diverse symptoms, but—as it would seem—permanently benefited by the propagation of lateral or transverse vibrations through the spinal column by the application of my percuteur to the ridge of the spinous processes. My method is to pass the percuteur slowly up and down the spine for ten minutes, or, if no disagreeable sensations are produced, a quarter of an hour, daily, or every second day. I believe the *modus operandi* of the treatment is to counteract the tendency to a lax and flaccid condition of the cord by exciting it to vibrate in a direction *at right angles* to its axis; most of the vibrations which act injuriously on the cord being propagated *in the line* of its axis. For the present I will simply make this statement, but I shall be glad to explain the matter more fully to any one who may be interested."

The publication of this letter excited a good deal of attention, and was the means of inducing many practitioners of repute to bring cases under my notice in consultation. A considerable proportion of these have subsequently been treated by nerve-vibration, with, I think I may say, generally good results. It is needless to chronicle the fact that there have been failures, but as the cases in which the treatment has been tried have been almost uniformly of the greatest gravity and long persistence, this is scarcely surprising.

INDIGESTION, CONSTIPATION, TENSION-ALBUMINURIA, AND PSEUDO-DIABETES.

Probably no such strange group of maladies was ever before made the subject of serious remark in a work designed exclusively for medical readers. Nevertheless, I venture to offer this grouping as a perfectly natural and scientific classification. Each and all of the disorders named are, in certain, at least, of their forms, due to nervous irritation, or nervous weakness; and it is maladies springing from these causes that I propose to treat by nerve-vibration.

First, there is a form of indigestion, and a very common one, too, which depends entirely on want of muscular movement in the stomach and intestines. The muscular fibres of the stomach do not act as they are intended to act, with a view to the turning over of the food in the organ and its admixture with the gastric secretion. Moreover, the absence of muscular movement and the deficiency of nerve power, leave the glands of the stomach without their natural mechanical stimulus to action and without energy, so that the secretion is insufficient in quantity, while its character is impaired. A special symptom of this condition, in which the organ more resembles a sac than a contractile organ, I have not seen mentioned in any work on medicine; albeit sufferers from this most troublesome form of dyspepsia commonly complain of it. They are unable to void the flatus with which the stomach becomes distended without making pressure on the epigastric region immediately below the sternum. The food taken into the stomach remains there until it undergoes much the same change that the maternal milk undergoes in the stomach of a weakly infant. It decomposes with the heat before it is so acted upon, in the process of digestion, as to be protected from the chemical and thermic influences that tend to decompose it. The stomach retains the food longer than is natural, and when at length it is extruded, or rather gravitates, through the pylorus into the duodenum and upper bowel, the time for intestinal digestion is passed. The action of the bowels in cases of this character is generally irregular, with a tendency to what is called "diarrhœa," having this characteristic, that the total amount passed is not large though defæcation occurs frequently, and the stools are patchy, consisting of portions of bilious fluid and imperfectly digested food. The matter voided tells the physiological story of the disease in a manner, which cannot be mistaken, if only the colour, consistency, and weight of the fæces receive the attention they deserve. The caput coli is nearly always distended in cases of this class, and it is often the seat of neuralgic pain.

I have lately seen some very striking examples of this muscular fault in digestion, and have found the effects of treatment by nerve-vibration to be exceedingly rapid and good. A very few days' percussion over the solar plexus has, first, relieved the inability to void flatus by the mouth, and then restored the natural action of the stomach with the result of putting an end to the whole trouble. The disturbance of, and pain in, the region of the colon has lingered somewhat, but within two or three weeks this too has yielded to treatment, and the patient has been not only relieved of his troubles, but found himself able to digest with entire comfort the very articles of food and drink which he did not previously dare to take. He has gained in weight. The stools have become natural, and the depressing effects of perpetual "bad digestion" have wholly disappeared. The flat-headed hammer or the hard brush serve the purpose well for the relief of this malady, and the result obtained is almost uniformly good and quickly gained, although the affection may have been the burden of life through long years. It will seem that I overstate the facts ; but the profession may readily put my assertions to the proof, and if cases be accurately diagnosed, I have no misgiving as to results.

For the treatment of constipation, by nerve-vibration

it is necessary to ascertain precisely where the fault lies. What is the cause of the retention of the fæces? What part of the intestinal canal fails in respect to the reflex by which the peristaltic movements are performed? In some instances the small intestines do not, so to say, feel the presence of the food *débris* above the ilio cæcal valve, with the effect of rendering the abdomen distended and dull on percussion, or dull and tympanitic in patches. In other cases the ascending colon is loaded, and a sense of weight, and often dragging pain are experienced in the right iliac fossa. Occasionally the transverse colon lies across the abdomen as a solid mass extending from right to left. In another variety of the affection the descending colon is loaded, and the rectum becomes filled with an indurated mass of fæces, the accumulation of many days. In a totally different class of cases the "constipation" is not caused by torpidity of the intestines, so much as by partial paralysis of the levator ani, and co-existing with this condition there is not unfrequently irritability of the sphincter, so that, although the lower bowel is loaded, there is no evacuation. The levator ani cannot draw up the anus. The attempt to do this immediately produces a strong contraction of the sphincter, so that only a thin squeezed morsel of the fæcal matter escapes.

Now, it is a curious and significant fact that vibration with my percuteur has never once, in my experience, produced peristaltic action! I believe the force of the blow is, under no circumstances, sufficient to accomplish that result, and here, as elsewhere, no effect whatever is produced by percussion over a muscle. If, however, the percuteur be applied with the flat-headed hammer over the lower dorsal, lumbar, and sacral, spines, and with the pointed ivory hammer, over the perineal nerves —striking these branches firmly—it is generally possible, in the course of a few days, to render the nerves so responsive, that the bowels act regularly, not be it observed, immediately after the nerve-vibration, but at the next habitual period. In only one instance have I known defæcation to occur soon after the percussion, and this was a case of locomotor ataxia. This effect followed the first administration of the vibration, and was not repeated, although the patient was under treatment for a month. The bowels acted regularly, or nearly so, every day, but not in any discernible relation to the remedy, so far as the immediate effects of vibration are concerned. I do not think it *possible* that so very slight a motion as is communicated by the percuteur, when most forcibly applied, can ever act on the bowels directly. It is only by reducing the nervous irritability, and heightening the response to the reflex generally, habitual constipation may be remedied. Employed or applied directly with the expectation of a speedy result, percussion cannot do otherwise than fail.

It is beginning to be recognized, but cannot yet be said to be commonly known, that albumen may and does appear in perfectly healthy urine, under conditions which either raise the tension of the blood in the vessels of the kidney to a very high point, or render the blood surcharged with albuminous material, as for example, when a patient lives almost exclusively on eggs. It is of course well-known that the urine often contains albumen during pregnancy, because the blood is then loaded with nutrient materials. It is, doubtless, similarly loaded immediately before each catamenial period, and, therefore, tension-albuminuria is physiologically likely to occur without any serious departure from the state of health at frequently recurring periods in the life of woman. The urine also contains albumen occasionally, soon after a heavy meal, or during particularly energetic muscular exertion, when the hard worker is also a voracious feeder and well supplied with albuminous food. Mere debility of the vessels of the kidney may allow the albumen to pass into the urine under these conditions. The systemic appetite seems to be over stimulated, so that more albumen is assimilated than the tissues require, and the surplusage is quickly thrown back into the current of the circulation, or passed off by the kidneys. Great and needless alarm is often caused by the discovery of albumen in the urine of young men who lead active lives, and particularly in that of brain-workers, who being overdone with intellectual labour resort to the unphysiological artifice of trying to work their bodies to relieve their minds, as though mind were something else than brain function, and the cerebrum was not an integral part of the organism as a whole. I have named this phenomenon *tension-albuminuria*, because it certainly needs to be known by some distinctive term if it is ever to be known at all; and looking to the misery inflicted on families by too hasty diagnoses and desperate prognoses which are not justified by the state or verified by the subsequent history of the case, it is time that an effort were made to secure the recognition of a "symptom" which does not necessarily indicate disease.

By pseudo-diabetes, I mean the presence of sugar in the urine with polyuria, or an increase in the quantity of urine passed on special occasions, with debility and wasting. The sugar is only found now and again, while the debility, which may be slight, or a serious feature of the case, is constant. The sugar appears when there is much irritation of the brain, and particularly when the "nervousness" is so great as to take the form of mental derangement, and render it difficult for the sufferer to mix in society, or even to sit in a room with his intimate friends. Toothache, or facial neuralgia, may accompany the malady, or there may be preternatural acuteness of hearing. I have seen several cases of this description recently, and in all it has been possible to trace the appearance of the sugar to special irritation of one of the nerves having a deep origin beneath the floor of the fourth ventricle. The "diabetes," falsely so called, is merely an incident in the course of another malady, which is generally neurosthenic in its type, and neurasthenic in its essential nature.

The treatment for tension-albuminuria and pseudo-diabetes, so far as nerve-vibration is concerned, is that which I have described for the various forms of neurasthenia, namely, percussion of the spinal column. The case of A. B., mentioned at page 107, may be cited as a good specimen of the class in which sugar is occasionally found in the urine. It is not by any means an uncommon thing to find sugar and albumen alternatively in the urine of ataxic or neurasthenic patients, more particularly, when great efforts are being made to struggle against the disease, and the sufferer, while undergoing much mental anxiety and taking a great deal of exercise, consumes a large quantity of stimulating food, under the impression that by a specially nourishing and full diet he may recover his failing strength. I think it is a condition of the appearance of the phenomenon that there should be an inordinate demand made by the organism, and more food assimilated than is required to replace the tissues consumed by use. We all recognize the existence of an organic appetite, distinct from the appetite or craving for food which proceeds from the stimulation of the nerves of taste or the unsatisfied longings of an empty stomach. This inner appetite is often more exigeant than the "appetite" properly so called. In the cases I am trying to indicate, I believe the inner, deeper, or organic appeal is itself exaggerated so that the tissues take up—or try to take up—more food than they require, and (if I may say so) dissimilation commences before assimilation is complete. Nerve-vibration seems to act in a very satisfactory way in these cases. It needs to be spinal in the main; but this general treatment should be supplemented by precise vibration of any of the nerves of special sense which may be found irritable, or of which the patient complains.

CONCLUSION.

I HAVE now briefly, and, I fear, very inadequately reviewed the leading points of the case I have to lay before the profession in support of my plea for nerve-vibration, at first, of course, in cases in which other remedies and methods of treatment have already been tried and failed. It is a severe but fitting ordeal through which any new therapeutic agent must pass, that it should be put to the test of being employed for the relief or cure of disorders which have been found to resist all the received modes of treatment. It is in such cases only, that I have yet myself employed nerve-vibration, and I shall be well content if others judge of its value by evidence collected on the same line of investigation. It would not be justifiable to omit or postpone recourse to such tried remedies as we already possess, but after all these are found to be useless, I venture to urge that the method I suggest should be accorded a trial.

In making choice of the several classes of cases in respect to which I now find myself in a position to recommend the use of nerve-vibration, I have been influenced solely by my experience of that remedy. I do not, because I cannot, strongly urge recourse to the method in a considerable number of troublous affections in the treatment of which I have not yet had any large experience of its use. Among these may be mentioned hysteria and the mimetic diseases, and disorders of the sexual organs, particularly impotence and the affection known, erroneously I believe, as spermatorrhœa. I have had cases of the two last-mentioned diseases, some of which have been and are, greatly benefited, one or two apparently cured, but a much larger number of observations than I have yet been able to make, would be necessary to justify any practitioner in holding out a hope that he had actually discovered a new remedy.

That the mimetic diseases may be successfully treated by nerve-vibration, I have little doubt; but I am not sure that any results gained in this department of therapy can be wholly trustworthy. In another group of affections in which I am much interested, I am hopeful that nerve-vibration may prove a valuable aid to other treatment, if not sufficiently good to stand alone, namely, the epileptic. The influence which precise nerve percussion undoubtedly exerts on the vaso-motor system certainly leads me to hope that the daily vibration of the anterior tibial nerve, or the corresponding nerve in the forearm will have a marked effect on the "fits." If this be not successful, I should vibrate the whole of the principal peripheral nerves with the brush or the disk, either applied directly to the skin or through water. I doubt whether it would be worth while to vibrate the solar plexus alone, but I should most certainly apply the flat-headed hammer or the hard brush over the epigastric region, alternately with the percussion over the anterior tibial nerve. In idiocy, even of the micro-cephalic type, I have already seen unmistakable proof of the efficacy of nerve-vibration as a means of rousing the dormant centres, and while effecting that immediate purpose, at the same time extending its influence to the improved nutrition of the body.

I have not seen any bad effects from nerve-vibration, and it is difficult to believe that, as it will be employed by medical practitioners, percussion with the very small and light instrument I use can possibly be harmful. The worst that is likely to happen is that, like most other methods of "cure," the new method may fail. There is one measure of treatment which I think nerve vibration should be allowed to precede, I refer to nerve-stretching. I do not think it is justifiable to undertake so formidable an operation as firmly stretching a nerve until so simple a remedy as nerve-vibration has been fairly and fully tried! The aim of the two specialties of treatment is unquestionably the same—namely, to change the character and rhythm of vibrations, which are either themselves painful, or induce the sensation of pain by the influence they exert on the vibration of other nerves. Nerve-stretching seeks to attain this object by the heroic expedient of stretching the nerve until its essential elements must be, for the time at least, thrown out of gear and mechanically disorganized. Nerve-vibration, on the other hand, makes the natural, and, it must be admitted, eminently rational endeavour to restore the discordant activity to order by the process whereby musical discords are silenced and concord is established. It may be urged that we stretch a violin or harp string to change the amplitude of its vibrations, and thus alter its tone, but the string of a musical instrument is not a living organ, and I think it will be conceded that we ought to try a perfectly harmless method of obtaining our object before we resort to one which, under the best circumstances, is formidable, and can never be justified until other means for the radical cure of the malady have been tried and proved of no avail.

I now leave this system of nerve-vibration in the hands of the medical profession, to be tried and either adopted or rejected, as it may prove deserving of either fate. For myself, I am fully persuaded that, whether or not my mode of applying the remedy is the best that can be devised, the underlying principle is sound, and the natural law I have sought to utilize is applicable to the relief of pain and the remedy of disease, and ought to be so employed.

THE END.

PRINTED BY BALLANTYNE, HANSON AND CO
LONDON AND EDINBURGH

Spotted something that isn't quite right?

Let us know and we'll fix it for future reprints. And as a thank you for your diligence, we'll send you a free Sothis book of your choice.

publisher@sothis.press

This page intentionally left blank

Except of course for that line above. And this one.
And whilst we have your attention, perhaps you'd
like to follow us on Instagram @sothis.press. Go on.

Made in United States
Orlando, FL
06 November 2026

90301618R00076